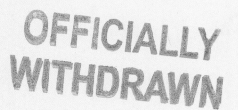
THE INVISION GUIDE TO

LIFEBLOOD

THE INVISION GUIDE TO

LIFEBLOOD

HarperCollins books may be purchased for educational, business, or sales promotional use. For information, please write: Special Markets Department, HarperCollins Publishers, 10 East 53rd Street, New York, NY 10022.

FIRST EDITION

Designed by Cindy Goldstein, assisted by Amy Wu,
Eric Baker Design Associates

Library of Congress Cataloging-in-Publication Data
has been applied for.

ISBN 978-0-06-087910-5

08 09 10 11 12/ QW 10 9 8 7 6 5 4 3 2 1

ACKNOWLEDGMENTS

Attila Ambrus, Chief Operating Officer:
For managing data acquisition, overall operations and always providing a reality check.

Matt Wimsatt, Director, Department of
Scientific Visualization:
For constant guidance, endless support and a calm demeanor primed to absorb the not-so-calm.

Laura Gibson, Project Manager:
For her inspiring versatility in management, conceptualization, research, writing, and editing. Her constant drive, painstaking attention to detail, devotion to content development and meticulous organization have laid the foundation for this book.

Jacquelyn Sun, Art Director:
For her keen eye, ability to conceptualize and actualize, unending patience, resiliency, and fluid manner with everyone on the team; for the perfect brainstorming and editing partner, and for her overall artistic drive.

Stephanie Allan, Project Manager Assistant:
For stepping in at a key time to help manage and expedite book content and spin-off projects.

Jeremy Mack, Creative Director/Photographer

Medical visualization specialists:
Stephanie Allan, Andres Arango, Ann Canapary, Laura Gibson, Ezra Kortz, Jeremy Mack, Mark Mallari, Chris Mendoza, Jean-Claude Michel, Gloria Situ, Shlomo Sam Spaeth, James Stanis, Jacquelyn Sun, Jessica Weisman, Matt Wimsatt, and Poy Yee, for their artistry, attention to detail, long hours, and individual and collective creativity.

Technical research and development specialists:
Laszlo Balogh, Chad Capeland, Matt Irwin, Ben Lipman

Photographers:
Jillian Cohen, Scott E. Moore, Jeremy Mack, Jacquelyn Sun

Designers:
Senior Designer Jacquelyn Sun and Associate Designer Poy Yee, for their creativity and design expertise.

Eric Baker Design, with special thanks to Eric Baker and Cindy Goldstein for their continued originality and ability to work under demanding deadlines.

Medical writers:
David Bjerklie, Margaret Blackstone, and Alice Park

Editors:
Stephanie Allan, David Bjerklie, Laura Gibson, Molly Lyons, Alice Park, Patrick Smith, and Jacquelyn Sun

Participating Anatomical Travelogue staff:
Sharon Ching, Stewart Deitch, Chin Huang, Ildiko McGivney and Danny Wong

Toni Sciarra at Collins:
For her patience and her thorough professionalism.

National Institutes of Health
National Library of Medicine and the Visible Human Project®

National Museum of Health and Medicine of the Armed Forces Institute of Pathology (AFIP)
Adrianne Noe, Director of the National Museum of Health and Medicine of the AFIP

Levine Plotkin & Menin, LLP and Bob Levine for his belief in our work and vision.

Photography credits:
Stock imagery is provided by the Science Source division of Photo Researchers Inc. (www.sciencesource.com)
Additional stock imagery obtained from Stock.XCHNG, p. 20-21

SEMS of hypertensive glomeruli from:
Stephen M. Bonsib, M.D., Albert G. and Harriet G. Smith Endowed Professor and Chair, Department of Pathology, Louisiana State University

© Leonid Mamchenkov, bowler, p. 52
© James Miller, chest X-ray, p. 56
© Brian Drake/Sports Illustrated, Sean Elliott, p. 86
© Michael Buckner/Corbis, George Lopez, p. 87
© Fortunato Amosco, kidney stone, p. 100
© D.B. King, cyclists, p. 104-105

Models:
Attila Ambrus, Junior Brown, Henry Kwok, Carson Kainer, Brandon Leslie, Adam Little, Jeremy Mack, Kent Moody and family, Tia Resan, Gloria Situ, Shlomo Sam Spaeth, James Stanis, James White, Stacy Young-Ripley

The individuals who graciously allowed us to share in and tell their stories:
Kent Moody, farmer, Crisman, Illinois
Brandon Leslie, professional runner, Albuquerque, New Mexico
Carson Kainer, baseball player, Dayton, Ohio

The crew of the Lifeblood documentary who made these stories possible:
Scott E. Moore, Director/Producer
Jillian Cohen, Associate Producer
Justine Angelis, Editor

Thanks also to Mark Liponis, M.D., Corporate Medical Director, Canyon Ranch, for sharing his story.

The imaging team at the Indiana Center for Biological Microscopy and staff at INPhoton, from whom we have learned much and with whom we hope to share many more years of collaboration. (http://www.inphoton.com)

The data specialists at Indiana University, whose skill and expertise with kidneys is unsurpassed:

Philip M. Blomgreen, M.S., Department of Anatomy, Indiana University School of Medicine

Kenneth Dunn, Ph.D., Associate Professor of Medicine, Scientific Director of Indiana Center for Biological Microscopy, Indiana University

Bruce Molitoris, M.D., Professor of Medicine, Director of Indiana Center for Biological Microscopy, Indiana University

Scientific advisors:

Carrie L. Phillips, M.D., Associate Professor of Medicine and Pathology, Specialist in Renal Pathology, Indiana University School of Medicine

Andy Evan, Ph.D., Professor of Anatomy and Cell Biology, Researcher of renal disease and pathology, Indiana University School of Medicine

Other specialists who have graciously shared their knowledge, time and advice:

Peter W. Marks, M.D., Ph.D., Associate Professor of Medicine, Specializing in Hematology, Yale University School of Medicine

Vincent H. Gattone II, Ph.D., Professor of Anatomy and Cell Biology, Indiana University School of Medicine

These individuals were instrumental in the accuracy and direction of the science and imagery that have pushed the limits of Anatomical Travelogue's skills and technology.

Roche, for providing the funding to produce these images. Special thanks to Chrys Kokino, for his professional support of this content.

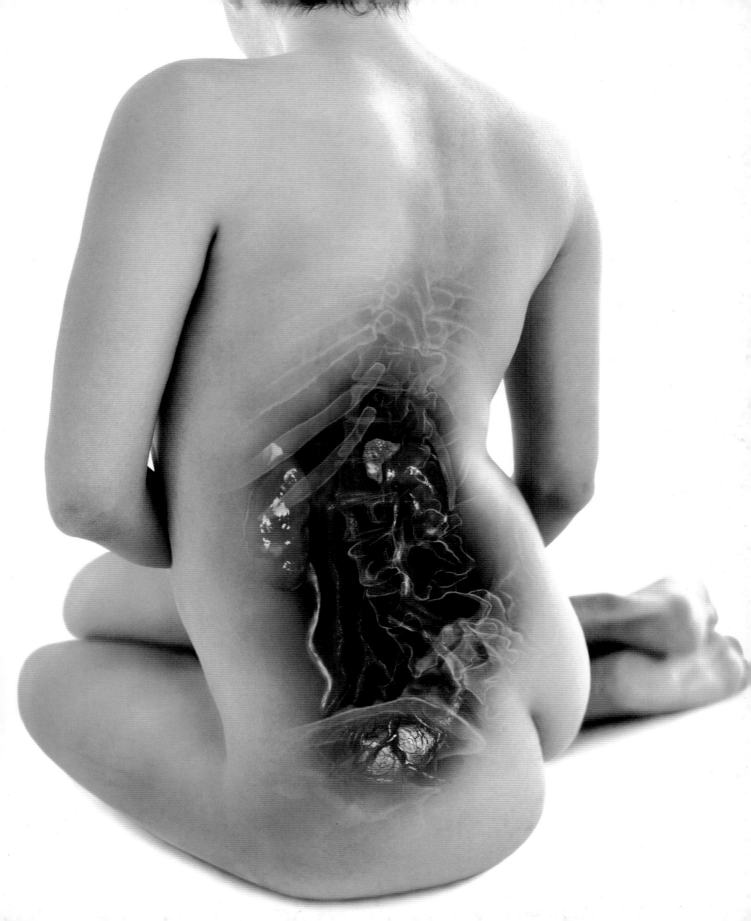

FOREWORD

In medical school I struggled with our nephrology course, the study of the kidneys. In many ways my kidneys seemed smarter than my poor overworked brain—able to perform so many vital functions with such perfection. Our kidneys are vital in regulating our blood pressure, fluid balance, pH buffering, blood formation, waste processing, and even our bone strength and bone health.

I remember spending many hours and late nights in the medical library studying mathematical formulas, trying to understand the function of the kidneys. Their anatomy was so complex and so beautiful; they seemed an engineering marvel. I could imagine a Lamborghini carburetor designer or a computer microchip engineer enviously trying to learn from the kidneys' miraculous construction and performance and hoping to gain insight or inspiration from the kidney.

I memorized the calculations for kidney function, filtration rates, and numerous mnemonics—memory tricks—to try and remember the many ways the kidneys could affect us in health and illness. I worried and fretted about the test questions that would inevitably appear on our exams and whether I would be able to come up with the right answers to these difficult questions.

But these lessons were nothing compared to the most personal nephrology lesson I could ever have—seeing and holding one of my own kidneys—in a jar in the pathology lab. My left kidney was removed 14 years ago, when I was 36 years old. What began as a minor nagging back pain that I attributed to being "middle-aged" declared itself with a single episode of blood in my urine that was soon diagnosed as a cancerous tumor. It's easier to talk about now, 14 years later, and I'm grateful for the success of surgery in removing this tumor that would otherwise undoubtedly have killed me.

But holding one of my own kidneys has had an indescribably powerful and yet ominous effect on me that has affected my life in so many profound ways. For the first time, I believe I truly appreciated the importance of the kidneys in health and longevity. I realized that my own kidney function had been acutely reduced by 50 percent, and I vowed to learn and to take steps to protect and preserve my remaining kidney.

I immediately went back to the books and began studying the kidneys again. Somehow it seemed clearer the second time around. I had a new focus, a new passion. The event was life-changing. I quit my job and began a preventive medicine practice to help teach people how to prevent disease, rather than experience the "wake-up call" that I had been through.

Over the past 14 years, not a day has gone by that I haven't appreciated the marvel of the kidneys and how critically important they are for our health. I thank the great designer who engineered them and who had the wisdom to provide us with two.

With my patients I spend a lot of time talking about the importance of our kidneys and how to protect and maintain their function. We test them and track their performance over time, making sure there is no decline in function. We carefully monitor blood pressure, red blood cell counts, hemoglobin, hematocrit, and creatinine, and repeatedly reinforce the importance of hydration—supplying the kidneys with adequate fluid to do their job and to perform optimally.

Of course I monitor my own kidney function and take steps to protect and preserve as much function as I possibly can. Since losing a kidney, I've become mildly anemic. As you'll learn by reading this wonderful book, that's no surprise. The kidneys are intimately involved in the formation of red blood cells.

I've also learned that with one remaining kidney, I need to take more vitamins—specifically more folic acid and B-complex vitamins. I need to eat more green,

leafy vegetables. And I need to take more vitamin D, an important vitamin for bone health that is also regulated by the kidneys. I also try to avoid eating too much protein—no more 16-ounce sirloins!

But most importantly, I've developed a deep and profound appreciation for the kidneys and their wide-ranging importance for our health. I continue to marvel at the kidneys' complexity and design. One of my goals is to try to convey to my patients how important it is to take care of their kidneys.

While reading and experiencing *The InVision Guide to Lifeblood*, I almost had a sense of déjà vu of when I held my own kidney in my hand—the images and explanations found in this book are so moving and powerful that I feel *Lifeblood* has the ability to inspire everyone to understand the vital nature and importance of our kidneys to our health and longevity. Please join me in experiencing, learning about, and protecting our precious kidneys!

Mark Liponis, M.D.,
Medical Director, Canyon Ranch

REVEALING THE BODY'S INNER MARVELS

The imagery in this book is the culmination of decades of effort to harness and hone the most advanced medical imaging technologies. The stunning visual results may look like the computer-generated graphics used in movies and video games. But in fact, the images in this book are of real cells, real vessels, tissues and organs. The visual data was collected in the course of medical evaluations with state-of-the-art medical imaging techniques, magnetic resonance imaging (MRI) and computerized tomography (CT).

How are these incredibly detailed images created? First, slices of tissue and organs are scanned layer by layer. The data from these two-dimensional snapshots are then analyzed and brought into focus. Next, the color in the images is enhanced where necessary to clearly show the boundaries of different cells and tissues. Data from the individual slices are re-assembled to build three-dimensional cells, tissues, organs and systems, as well as the pathologies that affect these systems. Hundreds or thousands of these individual slices are often needed to create a single organ.

The story the image can tell is further enhanced by the use of color, opacity and camera angle to either hide or highlight various elements—to look at red blood cells, for example, other cells and tissues can be stripped away for an unobstructed peek at only red blood cells in action. The final result is an unparalleled cell's-eye view of the body. These are the tools that are helping us to realize the dream of 16th-century anatomist Andreas Vesalius to reveal the workings of the body. Join us in this new "Fantastic Voyage" for the 21st century.

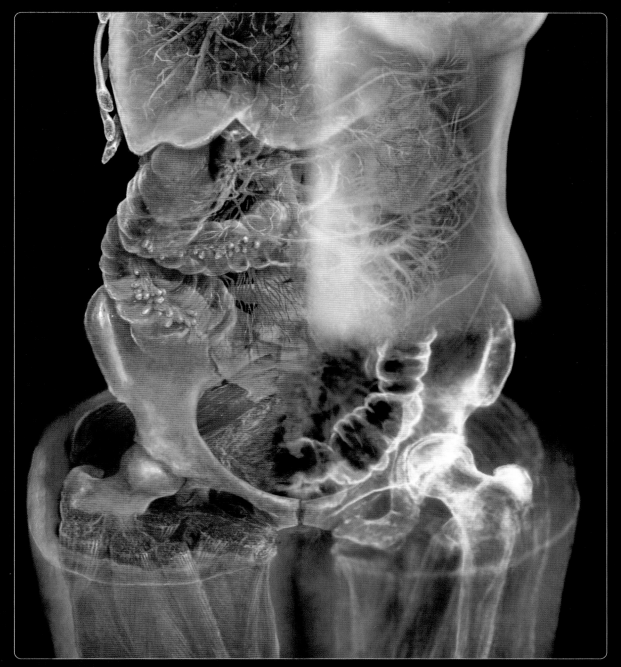

DIFFERENT SEGMENTATIONS AND RENDERING METHODS
APPLIED TO A COMPUTER TOMOGRAPHY (CT) DATASET

THE CAST
The kidneys, blood cells, stem cells and key molecules all play roles in a dynamic system that works to ensure your body's vitality.

THE KIDNEYS
Nestled in the small of the back, the kidneys are a pair of bean-shaped organs the size of a fist, located on each side of the spine, just below the rib cage. They are essential to the body's health because they filter wastes such as urea, toxins and excess salts out of the blood. Each day the kidneys filter 200 quarts of blood to produce about two quarts of waste and excess water as urine. They also play a critical role in maintaining the body's equilibrium by constantly adjusting the levels of key chemicals in the blood such as sodium, phosphorus and potassium. By increasing or decreasing the amount of salt and water the body excretes, the kidneys help to regulate blood pressure. And very importantly, they also monitor oxygen levels in the blood. If the kidneys detect an oxygen deficit, they respond by releasing the hormone erythropoietin (EPO).

THE RED BLOOD CELL (RBC)
The red blood cell is also called an erythrocyte: *erythro* is Greek for "red," *cyte* is Latin for "cell." The disc-shaped RBCs have the critical job of transporting oxygen from the lungs to the body's cells and bringing carbon dioxide from the cells back to the lungs to be expelled.

LIFEBLOOD'S ENSEMBLE

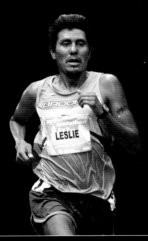

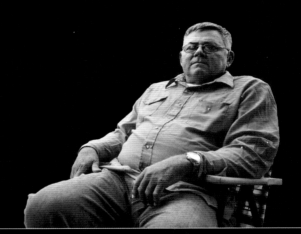

FULL OF ENERGY: BRANDON LESLIE
BRANDON LESLIE IS A PROFESSIONAL RUNNER. BRANDON'S TWO HEALTHY KIDNEYS AND BILLIONS OF RED BLOOD CELLS SUPPORT HIS TRAINING REGIMEN, WHICH INCLUDES RUNNING UP TO 20 MILES PER DAY., FULL OF ENERGY AND VITALITY, BRANDON IS A NATURAL COUNTERPOINT TO KENT MOODY, WHO SUFFERS FROM CHRONIC KIDNEY DISEASE AND ANEMIA.

FALLING ENERGY: KENT MOODY
KENT MOODY LOVES HIS FAMILY AND HE LOVES FARMING. FOR YEARS, WITH THE SUPPORT OF HIS FAMILY AND DOCTORS, HE HAS BEEN ABLE TO MANAGE HIS DIABETES AND HYPERTENSION AND CONTINUE FARMING THE LONG 12-18 HOUR DAYS. BUT OVER THE YEARS, BOTH DISEASES HAVE TAKEN THEIR TOLL ON KENT'S KIDNEYS. KENT SUFFERS FROM CHRONIC KIDNEY DISEASE (CKD) AND ACCOMPANYING ANEMIA. IN THIS BOOK, YOU WILL BE ABLE TO SHARE IN KENT'S PATHWAY TO HEALTH AS HE STRUGGLES TO OVERCOME CKD AND ANEMIA AND FINALLY EMERGES WITH A NEW KIDNEY, COMPLETELY REVITALIZED.

HEMOGLOBIN

Hemoglobin is an iron-rich protein that is packed inside RBCs. It is a structurally complex molecule that can change shape to either hold or release oxygen, depending on the body's need. Each RBC contains close to 300 million hemoglobin molecules.

STEM CELLS

Stem cells can give rise to a large number of specialized blood cells, including RBCs. Pluripotent hematopoietic stem cells are the progenitor cells from which all blood cells originate. *Hemat* is Latin and Greek for "blood," *poiesis* is Greek for "creation," and *pluripotent* is Latin for "capable of being many things." It is the hormone EPO which is released from the kidneys, that instructs a cell derived from a stem cell to become a RBC. (Technically, the cell that EPO binds to is called a stem/progenitor cell, but we will refer to it in this book as simply a stem cell).

OXYGEN

Oxygen enters the body with each breath and spread through the lungs' vast network of tiny air sacs an capillaries, where it can then enter the bloodstrear There, millions of hemoglobin molecules in the RBC grab onto the oxygen molecules and escort them a the RBCs travel through the body. As the RBCs pas by cells that need oxygen, hemoglobin changes i shape in order to release oxygen molecules, whic then pass through blood vessel walls and into th cells that will use the oxygen to convert nutrients int energy.

ERYTHROPOIETIN (EPO)

Bringing together the Greek words *erythro*, for "red and *poiesis*, for "creation," EPO is true to its nam this hormone, a chemical messenger produced in th kidneys, travels to the bone marrow where it orches trates one of the body's vital functions—initiating th creation of red blood cells.

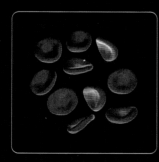

RED BLOOD CELL

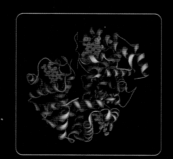

HEMOGLOBIN

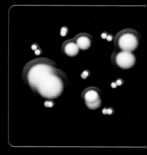

OXYGEN

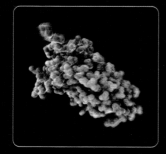

ERYTHROPOIETIN

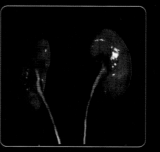

KIDNEYS

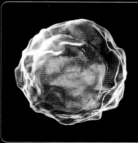

STEM CELL

our blood is the river of life. It ferries oxygen through a vast network of vessels and capillaries to every cell of your body, from your brain to your big toe. But the blood could not supply the body with oxygen without the help of the kidneys.

Why are healthy RBCs dependent on healthy kidney function? Because the kidneys produce EPO, the essential hormone that flips the on-switch for RBC production from the bone marrow's stem cells. The kidneys also cleanse the blood of the cellular waste products the body has collected. The constant cycling of the blood through the kidneys keeps the blood balanced so that it, in turn, can keep the body functioning optimally.

Lifeblood is the story of how the kidneys perform their critical role in maintaining vitality and blood balance and what happens when they can no longer do so. When chronic kidney disease (CKD) develops, this exquisite equilibrium is compromised and chronic anemia results. The goal of *Lifeblood* is to explain the underlying causes of chronic illness and to guide individuals toward achieving and maintaining a life of energy and vigor.

PERFECT PARTNERS: BLOOD AND KIDNEYS

1

A Welcome Population Boom
On average, a person has 20 to 30 trillion red blood cells coursing through his or her blood vessels (men actually have a few billion more than women). This means you have more red blood cells at work in your body than there are stars in the Milky Way.

55% PLASMA

<1% WHITE BLOOD CELLS
<1% PLATELETS

45% RED BLOOD CELLS

THE VITAL
COMPONENTS
OF BLOOD

55% PLASMA

Plasma is the liquid river that transports every blood cell to its destination. Oxygen-carrying RBCs couldn't move through arteries, veins and capillaries without it. Even though it is a watery, almost clear fluid, plasma contains many important substances, including blood-clotting agents called platelets and protective proteins called antibodies which help us fight infection. When the clotting agents are removed from blood plasma, it is called serum, which is essential in many life-saving medical situations such as transplant surgery and trauma.

<1% WHITE BLOOD CELLS
(WBCS OR LEUKOCYTES)

Some leukocytes are produced in the bone marrow, while others are generated in lymph nodes scattered throughout the body. They are far less numerous than their sister RBCs, but leukocytes are the bedrock of the immune system and are the body's front line of defense. Different types of leukocytes fight infections in different ways. Some target bacterial or fungal infections, while others respond to parasitic threats or allergic reactions.

<1% PLATELETS

Platelets perform the vital function of clotting blood at wound sites. They are small, even in comparison to the other cells of your blood, but they pack a wallop when it comes to healing a scrape or staunching a more serious wound. When you cut yourself shaving, platelets arrive on the scene like your personal emergency medical team, creating a natural bandage of clotted blood, which eventually forms a scab.

45% RED BLOOD CELLS
(RBCS OR ERYTHROCYTES)

RBCs are produced in the bone marrow and perform the fundamental task of delivering oxygen to all of the body's cells.

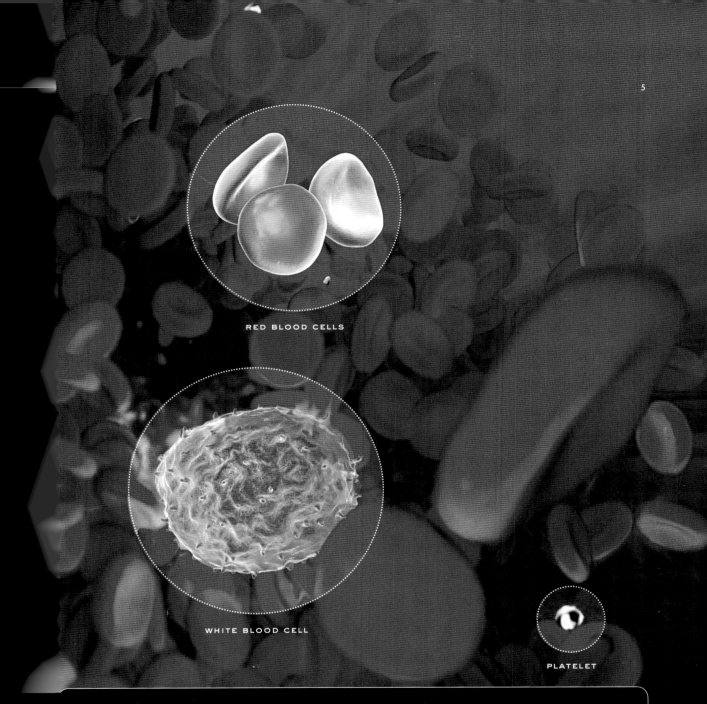

RED BLOOD CELLS

WHITE BLOOD CELL

PLATELET

HEMATOCRIT AND HEMOGLOBIN: THE ESSENTIAL TOOLS IN DIAGNOSING ANEMIA

The hematocrit is one of many tests that make up the complete blood count (CBC). Hematocrit measures the volume of RBCs in your blood. A normal hematocrit reading for women is between 36 to 44 percent; for men it's 41 to 50 percent.

The hemoglobin test measures the amount of hemoglobin molecules in the blood. A normal range is around ⅓ the hematocrit: 12 to 15 gm/dL in women and 13 to 17 gm/dL in men.

If your readings for hematocrit and hemoglobin are below these ranges, you may be at risk for or already have anemia.

MAKING BLOOD: FROM STEM CELLS TO RED BLOOD CELLS

The creation of RBCs requires the physiological marriage of the kidney and the stem cell. Think of the kidney as the "father," the stem cell as the "mother" and EPO as the "sperm" sent by the father through the bloodstream to inseminate the stem cell, which then goes on to manufacture millions of RBC "progeny."

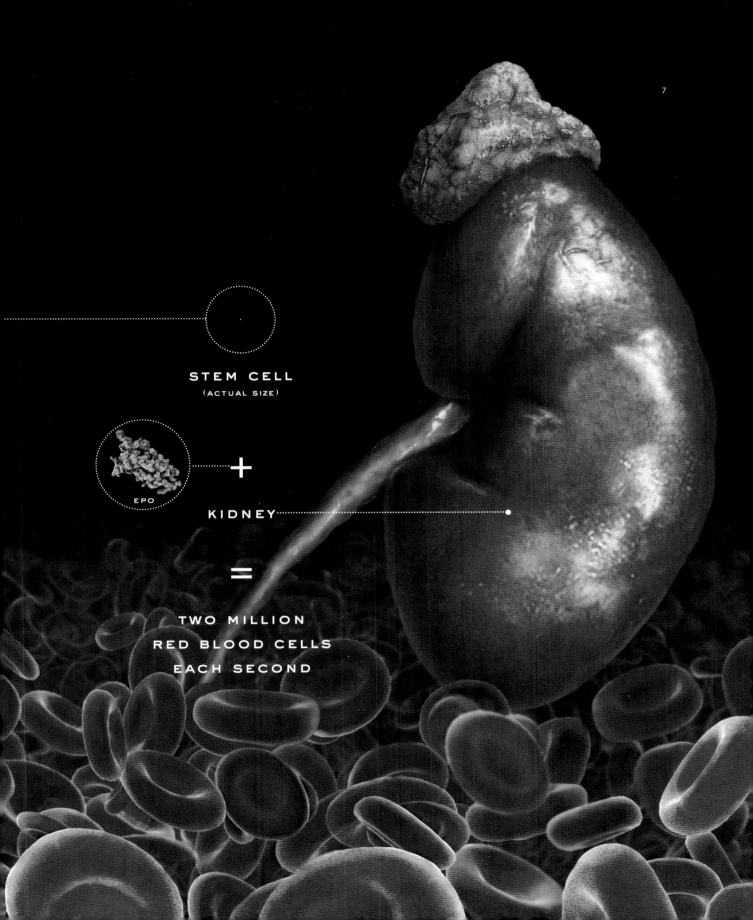

STEM CELL
(ACTUAL SIZE)

EPO

+

KIDNEY

=

TWO MILLION
RED BLOOD CELLS
EACH SECOND

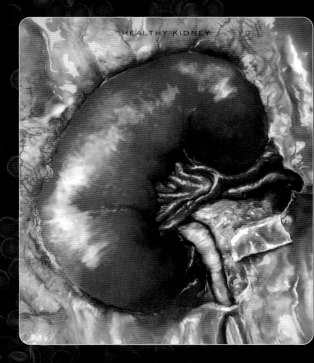

HEALTHY KIDNEY

THE CONNECTION:
CKD AND
CHRONIC ANEMIA

Chronic kidney disease (CKD) results when the kidneys are increasingly unable to balance adequate levels of electrolytes (like sodium or calcium) and fail to produce enough urine to eliminate the toxins and other waste from the bloodstream. Twenty million Americans, or one in nine adults, have CKD and 20 million more are at risk. At present CKD is the ninth leading cause of death in the U.S. Globally, more than 500 million individuals, or about one in 10 adults, have some degree of CKD. CKD contributes to the deaths of over 12 million individuals worldwide each year—a number that is rapidly increasing.

When kidney function declines, kidney cells die too, which further compromises the critical role the organ plays in RBC development, balancing electrolytes and filtering wastes. The deterioration of kidney func-

tion leads to further deterioration in the organ. It is easy to see how CKD can get progressively worse until the organ just shuts down.

Most cases of CKD unfold over years and even decades. The fact that it can develop gradually and with few or no symptoms in the early stages makes it an especially insidious threat. The major enemies of kidney health in developed countries are diabetes and hypertension, both of which are tied to overall precarious health, poor diet and obesity. In fact, diabetes and hypertension are responsible for 65 percent of cases of CKD.

There are many other medical problems that can compromise your kidney function. An accident or direct trauma to the kidney can cause acute kidney failure. So can infections that directly injure the kidney or a severe

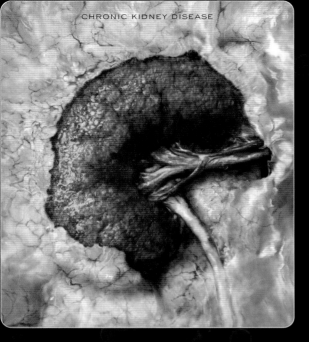

illness that is accompanied by dehydration, nausea and vomiting. Long-term use of pain medications, such as non-steroidal anti-inflammatory agents like acetaminophen and ibuprofen and certain enzyme inhibitors may also tax the organ and cause CKD. Other causes of CKD include infections that spread through the blood, certain antibiotics, lead poisoning, an enlarged prostate gland or an inherited DNA mutation causing kidney malfunction.

Kidney damage can easily go unnoticed until the situation is serious and kidneys are working at just 15 percent of their normal capacity. Most cases of CKD, in fact, are diagnosed when there is already irreversible kidney damage.

When symptoms do occur in acute kidney failure, they may include:

• swelling of the feet and ankles

• sudden decrease in urination

• loss of appetite accompanied by nausea or vomiting

• muscle cramps and twitches

• malaise and/or drowsiness

In chronic kidney failure, additional symptoms may include:

• metallic taste in the mouth, an "acid" smell in breath, and hiccups because of the buildup of waste in the bloodstream

• itching due to high phosphorus levels

• mental dullness or lack of acuity because of inadequate oxygen delivery to brain cells

If the kidney does not respond to treatment, the result is CKD. And because CKD affects the production of EPO, and thus RBC production, anemia almost always precedes or accompanies a diagnosis of CKD.

Anemia is caused when there are too few RBCs circulating in the bloodstream. That can happen when they are lost through bleeding, destroyed too quickly or produced too slowly. Anemia can also be caused by deformed RBCs, which is the case in inherited sickle cell anemia, or when the cells are either too large or too small to function properly.

When a person is anemic, the blood cannot do an effective job of transporting the oxygen inhaled from the lungs to all the tissues of the body. Anemic blood is also less effective in retrieving carbon dioxide from the tissues and carrying it back to the lungs to be exhaled. The blood simply cannot do its job as well as it should. The old expression "tired blood" is an apt one.

In most cases, anemia is a secondary condition caused by an underlying disease, but it can also be a primary disease itself, such as sickle cell anemia, an inherited disorder. And like kidney disease, anemia

VITALITY GAINED

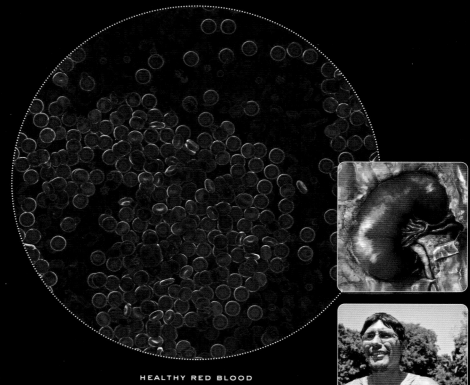

HEALTHY RED BLOOD
CELL COUNT

Runner Brandon Leslie has healthy kidneys and therefore has a healthy amount of RBCs that deliver oxygen to his body, supplying energy and enabling him to run at peak performance.

can be chronic, a condition that develops and persists over a long period of time. In some cases, however, it can be acute, brought on more rapidly by abnormal blood loss, or by an illness like cancer or even by medical treatments such as chemotherapy or radiation therapy.

There are many different types of anemia and their symptoms will vary by type and also vary in severity. Some of the most common symptoms, espe-

cially for the chronic anemia that accompanies include shortness of breath and loss of energy, [diz]ness, loss of appetite and weight loss, joint ten[der]ness and coldness or numbness in the hands or [feet]. Pale skin is also often a sign. But pallor alone[,] dizziness or appetite, isn't necessarily definitive. [Skin] tone is affected by several factors. Someone [with] even severe anemia, for example, might still [blush] when embarrassed.

VITALITY LOST

ANEMIC RED BLOOD
CELL COUNT

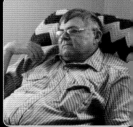

Farmer Kent Moody has diseased kidneys and therefore has a low, unhealthy amount of RBCs that are unable to deliver the necessary amount of oxygen to is body, consequently causing his fatigue

THE HUMAN BODY RUNS ON JUST
FIVE LITERS OF BLOOD. THAT'S
ABOUT A GALLON PLUS A QUART.

2

IN SYNC:
WHEN BLOOD
AND THE KIDNEYS
WORK TOGETHER

The kidneys and the blood efficiently nourish cells and remove wastes. In this chapter we'll look at the healthy workings of this elegant and essential partnership in action.

BRANDON LESLIE'S BODY IS PERFORMING AT PEAK ABILITY, ENABLING HIM TO SUPPLY CONSTANT ENERGY THROUGHOUT HIS BODY FOR HOURS AT A TIME.

A RUNNER'S HIGH

There is no better example of the perfect balance between the kidneys and the blood than the body of an athlete. Brandon Leslie, a professional marathon runner training for the 2008 Olympic marathon, doesn't spend much time thinking about blood cells or filtration rates, but he does know that his kidneys need to be in peak condition if he is going to push his body to perform.

Leslie's body wasn't always in such great shape. As a Native American who spent his vacations and weekends on a reservation in New Mexico, Leslie showed an early talent for running, but college proved too distracting and disorienting. At 19 he learned that he would be a father, and dropped out of school, only returning several years later. Finally, deciding that he needed to support his family, he gave up running altogether and took a job. Like his father before him, he began drinking heavily and gained 20 pounds. "I still had dreams of wanting to run professionally but I had doubts because I started living the life of just working, eating, going out, and living the nightlife on weekends." Finally, after meeting his current wife Nelvina, Leslie decided he did not want to be another Native American athlete who gave up. "That's what happens to a lot of Native American athletes; they have so much talent but they don't continue because of a bad decision, and I wanted to show people that it's possible to overcome failures and to overcome obstacles."

Today, Leslie takes advantage of his upbringing in the high altitude of Gallup, New Mexico. After a trip to a sea-level event in Florida, he realized that his training in thinner air gives him an advantage in endurance and strength at sea level. "It was weird because I wondered why am I running this fast and not struggling to gasp for oxygen or feeling so tired," he says. "It was just really easy. And the recovery was really quick."

What was happening was that having been born and raised at 5,000 feet above sea level, his body had become adjusted, or acclimatized, to the reduced amounts of oxygen in the air there. His RBCs pick up less oxygen, which means his muscles receive less oxygen, making it harder to keep them working. In response, his kidneys start to churn out more EPO, which in turn produces more RBCs to try to suck more oxygen from the air.

So when he runs at low altitude, his body has literally been physiologically primed, stocked with more RBCs capable of feeding oxygen to his muscles. This is what allows him to run faster, feel better, and recover more quickly. He's a perfect model for how efficient the body's kidneys and blood system can be – and an ideal role model for the Navajo Nation. "I hope I can show people that you can overcome [your failures]. You just have to put your mind and your heart into it."

AN EXQUISITE MODEL OF FORM AND FUNCTION

A single drop of blood contains roughly five million RBCs. Blood cells are minuscule and yet it is precisely their small size that allows them to accomplish their enormous tasks so effectively. The RBC is disc-shaped and concave on both sides. Imagine a tiny, cookie-shaped piece of dough that you squeeze between your thumb and forefinger. It is a form that's uniquely adapted to the RBCs' function.

The concave shape increases the cells' surface area, which allows them to distribute more oxygen to the body's cells. The shape also enables the cells to bunch together more compactly, helping them travel through the bloodstream more efficiently. Some RBCs are a bit thicker or thinner, wider or longer than others, but can change their shape to suit the demands of their environment. The cell membranes of the RBCs are protein meshes that give them flexibility, allowing them to navigate the twists and turns of the blood vessel network. The nearly 300 million hemoglobin molecules contained within each RBC easily move and slide past each other within the cell, adjusting their positions to conform to the RBC's shifting shape.

THE RED BLOOD CELLS' ABILITY TO BEND AND FLEX DUE TO THE STRUC-TURE OF THEIR MEMBRANES HELPS THEM TO SURVIVE AS THEY COURSE THROUGH TORTUOUS BLOOD VESSELS.

THE RED BLOOD CELL CONSISTS OF A SPONGE-LIKE, PROTEIN-RICH FRAME. THIS FRAME HOUSES HEMOGLOBIN MOLECULES. THE REST OF THE CELL IS COMPOSED OF FATTY SUBSTANCES THAT SUPPORT HEMOGLOBIN PRODUCTION.

HEMOGLOBIN, THE RED BLOOD CELLS' BRILLIANT CONTRIBUTION

Hemoglobin is the protein that is responsible for carrying oxygen in the RBC. It's composed of four smaller proteins called "globins." Each of the four globins holds onto a molecule called a "heme." An iron atom, the essential ingredient for oxygen binding, is cradled and protected by each of the four heme molecules. Each hemoglobin molecule is therefore capable of binding four oxygen molecules. When oxygen binds to the iron atom within the heme group, the RBC and blood itself turns red in color.

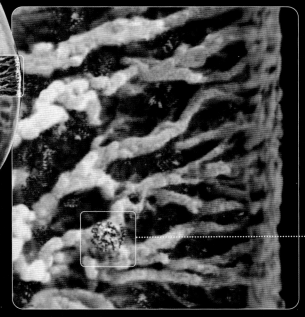

THE PROTEIN MESH OF A RED BLOOD CELL MEMBRANE

HEMOGLOBIN

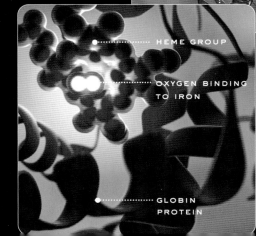

HEME GROUP

OXYGEN BINDING TO IRON

GLOBIN PROTEIN

A HEME GROUP CONSISTS OF AN IRON ATOM BOUND EQUALLY TO FOUR NITROGEN ATOMS. ALL LYING IN ONE PLANE. THE IRON ATOM IS THE SITE OF OXYGEN BINDING.

THE BREATH
OF LIFE

Red blood cells are responsible for delivering oxygen to all the cells and tissues of the body and for clearing away carbon dioxide and other wastes. When we inhale, oxygen and other gases travel through the nasal or oral cavities, then to the pharynx and down the trachea and into either the left or right bronchi to the lungs. There, oxygen passes through the porous walls of tiny air sacs called alveoli, where it enters the blood through the surrounding capillaries. After the RBCs deliver the oxygen to the body's tissues, they pick up carbon dioxide and carry it back to the lungs where the process is reversed and the carbon dioxide is expelled when we exhale. This miracle of molecular transportation is performed with each of the roughly 20,000 breaths we take every day.

RED BLOOD CELLS CARRY OXYGEN TO MUSCLES AND OTHER TISSUES.

THE COMPOSITION OF AIR
As essential as it is, oxygen comprises only 20 percent of the air we breathe. The other components are nitrogen (78.08 percent), argon (0.93 percent) and carbon dioxide (0.038 percent).

THE OXYGEN DELIVERY CYCLE

WITHIN THE LUNGS OXYGEN FLOWS INTO AN ALVEOLAR SAC.

TRACHEA

LUNG

RED BLOOD CELLS PICK UP OXYGEN IN THE ALVEOLAR CAPILLARIES. THIS IS WHEN THEY TURN BRIGHT RED.

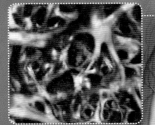

BONE MARROW

RED BLOOD CELL

KIDNEY

THE LIFE AND DEATH OF A RED BLOOD CELL

Our RBCs are not immortal, but their production continues throughout our lifetime, thanks to the constantly renewing stem cells in our bone marrow.

In the blood of a healthy individual, about 2.5 million RBCs are destroyed every second. But luckily that's (quite literally) less than a drop in the bucket, since we have a total of 20 to 30 trillion RBCs in the body. Still, to maintain the body's healthy equilibrium, the RBCs must be replaced constantly.

In the first weeks of embryonic development, RBCs are created by stem cells that grow in the yolk sac along with the fetus. Beginning at the third month of gestation, both the developing liver and spleen start to contribute to the stem cell and RBC pool. By the fifth month bone marrow has developed and your bones become the dominant production sites for stem cells, the biological factories for future blood cells.

Throughout childhood the marrow in all bones contain stem cells that can in turn produce RBCs and other blood components. But as kids mature into adults, the creation of RBCs is mostly restricted to the marrow from the ends of the "long" bones—the vertebrae, ribs, and pelvis—with a little produced in the skull. In the case of severe illness or accident, the marrow within the entire leg and arm bones may be called back into service temporarily.

The life cycle of a normal RBC is about 120 days, just four months. But in that short lifetime the RBC makes an astonishing 75,000 round trips between the lungs, heart and cells of the body. Since RBCs do not possess a nucleus, they are unable to repair or synthesize new cellular components. So eventually they wear out.

When that happens, most aging RBCs are pulled out of circulation by specialized white blood cells called macrophages within the liver, spleen, and lymph nodes. The macrophages engulf RBCs, "digest" them and release some of their components to be recycled within the body.

One of the components, iron, the bloodstream's precious metal, is neither destroyed nor eliminated, but is instead constantly reused to bind oxygen over and over. As soon as the aging and damaged RBCs are dismantled, the iron is picked up by newly formed RBCs in need of an iron atom. This explains why, though we do need iron in our diet, we need only small quantities of it. Our body naturally keeps a ready supply on hand.

At the same time that old RBCs are broken down and their components re-utilized, the bone marrow is at work producing new RBCs. In a healthy human being, this is a dynamic and continuous process.

LIVER   SPLEEN

MACROPHAGES IN THE SPLEEN AND THE LIVER WEED OUT OLD AND DEFECTIVE RED BLOOD CELLS AND BREAK THEM INTO RECYCLABLES (IRON, HEME, AND SOME GLOBIN) AND WASTES (SUCH AS BILIRUBIN).

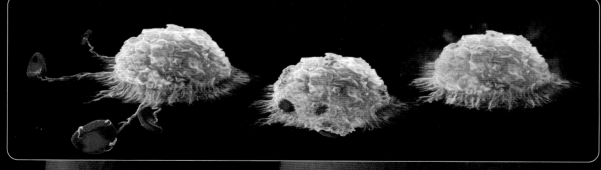

CAPTURE   ENGULF   RECYCLE

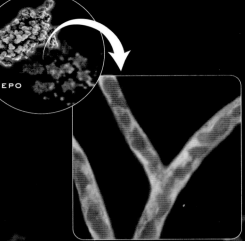

EPO

THE BLOOD AND KIDNEYS ARE INTIMATELY
CONNECTED BY EPO. WHEN LOW OXYGEN
LEVELS ARE DETECTED IN THE BLOOD AS IT
TRAVELS THROUGH THE KIDNEYS, THESE
MASTERS OF BALANCE PRODUCE EPO. ONCE
THE STEM CELLS IN THE BONE MARROW
RECEIVE THIS MESSAGE FROM THE KIDNEYS,
THEY BEGIN TO PRODUCE RED BLOOD CELLS.

CLOSE-UP
INTERLOBULAR
ARTERIES

INTERLOBULAR
ARTERIES

ARCUATE
ARTERIES

ARCUATE ARTERIES BRANCHING
INTO INTERLOBULAR ARTERIES

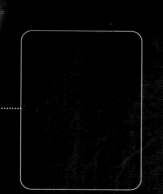

KIDNEYS: THE BLOOD'S RECYCLING CENTER

Blood cycles through the dense capillary forests in the kidneys up to 400 times a day. The kidneys are engaged in a dynamic, open dialogue with the blood, and are constantly adjusting levels of key substances, depending on what the body needs.

The kidneys are the body's primary filtering system, responsible for processing and eliminating wastes from the bloodstream such as excess salts and proteins. Once extracted, these are then broken down into a substance called urea. Urea flows to the bladder and is eventually expelled as urine.

Working non-stop day and night, the kidneys filter nearly 200 quarts of blood per day, producing about two quarts of urine (depending on body size). But that's just the beginning of the critical functions the kidneys perform.

OUR BODY'S TIRELESS FILTER

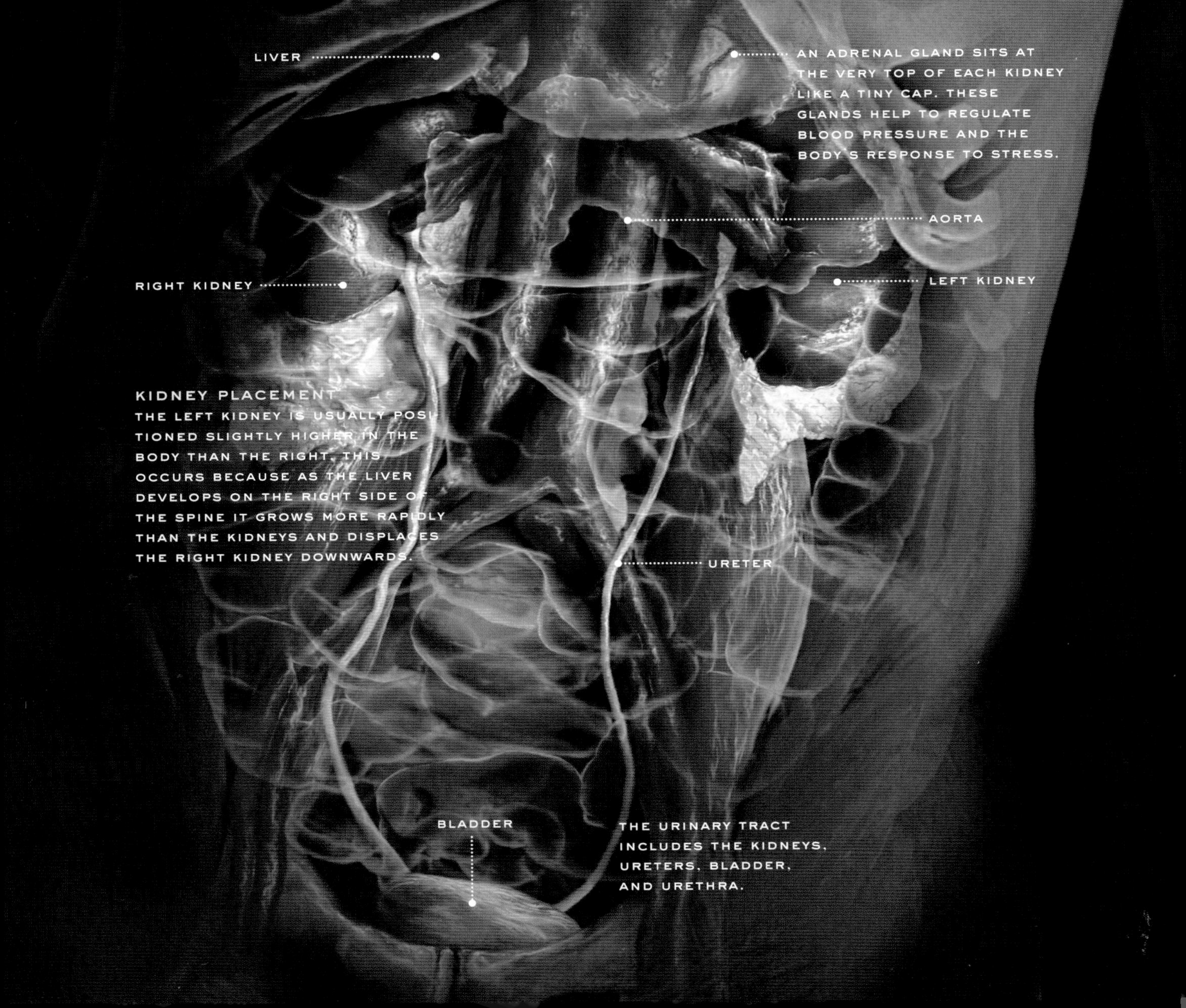

LIVER

AN ADRENAL GLAND SITS AT THE VERY TOP OF EACH KIDNEY LIKE A TINY CAP. THESE GLANDS HELP TO REGULATE BLOOD PRESSURE AND THE BODY'S RESPONSE TO STRESS.

AORTA

RIGHT KIDNEY

LEFT KIDNEY

KIDNEY PLACEMENT
THE LEFT KIDNEY IS USUALLY POSITIONED SLIGHTLY HIGHER IN THE BODY THAN THE RIGHT. THIS OCCURS BECAUSE AS THE LIVER DEVELOPS ON THE RIGHT SIDE OF THE SPINE IT GROWS MORE RAPIDLY THAN THE KIDNEYS AND DISPLACES THE RIGHT KIDNEY DOWNWARDS.

URETER

BLADDER

THE URINARY TRACT INCLUDES THE KIDNEYS, URETERS, BLADDER, AND URETHRA.

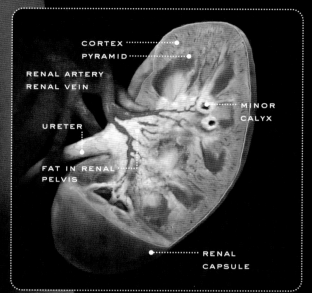

CORTEX

PYRAMID

RENAL ARTERY
RENAL VEIN

URETER

FAT IN RENAL
PELVIS

MINOR
CALYX

RENAL
CAPSULE

BLOOD FLOWS IN THROUGH THE RENAL ARTERY,
ENDING UP IN THE CORTEX OF THE KIDNEYS,
WHERE THE FILTERING PROCESS TAKES PLACE.
THE FILTRATE, WHICH INCLUDES WASTES REMOVED
FROM THE BLOOD, PASSES THROUGH TUBULAR
NETWORKS AND IS FUNNELED DOWN FROM
THE PYRAMIDS TO THE CALYCES TO THE RENAL
PELVIS, WHERE THE URETER CARRIES THE FLUID
OUT OF THE KIDNEY. THE URINE FLOWS FROM THE
URETER TO THE BLADDER, WHERE IT IS STORED
UNTIL READY FOR RELEASE VIA THE URETHRA.

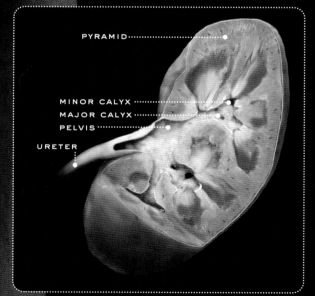

PYRAMID

MINOR CALYX
MAJOR CALYX
PELVIS

URETER

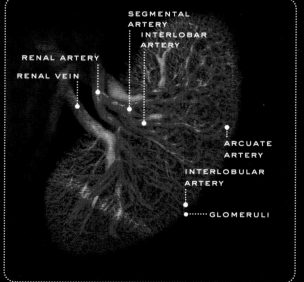

SEGMENTAL
ARTERY
INTERLOBAR
ARTERY

RENAL ARTERY

RENAL VEIN

ARCUATE
ARTERY

INTERLOBULAR
ARTERY

GLOMERULI

WHAT HAPPENS WHEN KIDNEYS FALTER

The kidneys perform one of the finest balancing acts found in nature. The relative acidity or alkalinity of a liquid is measured as its pH. To be healthy, our bodies demand that the blood stays within a narrow range of pH, slightly alkaline, but close to neutral. The kidneys help the blood to maintain its equilibrium by providing a buffer solution—one that will compensate for any rise or fall in levels of acid or base caused by diet or stress. The kidneys accomplish this balancing act by adjusting the amount of fluids and vital salts, called electrolytes, in your blood. The electrolytes include sodium, potassium, calcium and other substances needed to maintain a steady pH.

In addition your kidneys function as glands, producing two vital hormones: renin, which helps to control blood pressure, and EPO, which stimulates RBC production in the bone marrow and plays a key role in helping to maintain oxygen levels in the blood. As if this were not enough, your kidneys also manufacture the active form of vitamin D, which aids in monitoring the amount of calcium in the body, keeping your bones healthy.

BACK OR FLANK PAIN
IRREGULAR HEARTBEAT
KIDNEY STONES
EXCESSIVE THIRST
HIGH BLOOD PRESSURE

CALCIUM (EXCESS)

+

EXCESS

−

DEFICIENCY

CALCIUM (DEFICIENCY)

MUSCLE SPASMS
TINGLING FINGERS AND TOES
MENTAL CONFUSION
WEAK HEART CONTRACTIONS

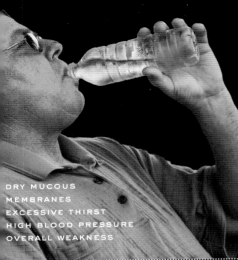

DRY MUCOUS
MEMBRANES
EXCESSIVE THIRST
HIGH BLOOD PRESSURE
OVERALL WEAKNESS

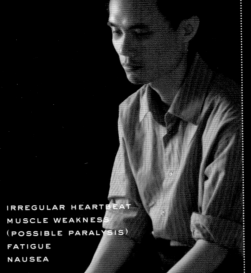

IRREGULAR HEARTBEAT
MUSCLE WEAKNESS
(POSSIBLE PARALYSIS)
FATIGUE
NAUSEA

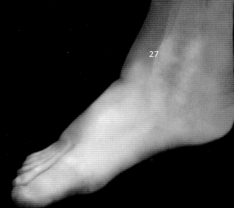

HIGH BLOOD PRESSURE
EDEMA

SODIUM

POTASSIUM

RENIN

HYPERTENSIVE KIDNEY

SODIUM

POTASSIUM

CALCITROL

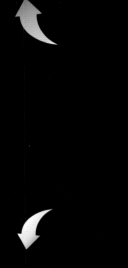

MUSCLE CRAMPS
FATIGUE
ABDOMINAL DISCOMFORT
AND CRAMPS
HEADACHE AND NAUSEA
SEIZURES

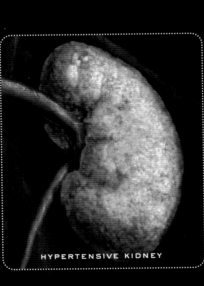

IRREGULAR HEARTBEAT
MUSCLE WEAKNESS
FEELING OF PINS AND NEEDLES
IN EXTREMITIES
DECREASED APPETITE
FREQUENT URINATION

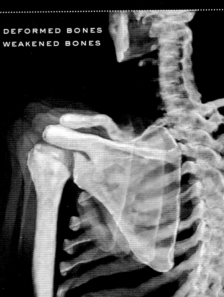

DEFORMED BONES
WEAKENED BONES

FROM THE INSIDE OUT: ANOTHER PERSPECTIVE ON THE KIDNEYS

The kidneys are located on each side of the spine, just below the ribcage and toward the back of the body, below the liver and the spleen. Each is about the size of a fist. A cushioning fat pad protects them along with the sheets of muscle that support your back and help to shield these highly complex organs from injury.

While biology provides us with two kidneys, one healthy kidney is perfectly capable of doing the whole job.

MUSCLE TISSUE
PROTECTS THE KIDNEYS

KIDNEY

RIB

PERIRENAL
FAT

A FIBROUS CAPSULE
FURTHER INSULATES
THE KIDNEY FROM HARM

SPINE

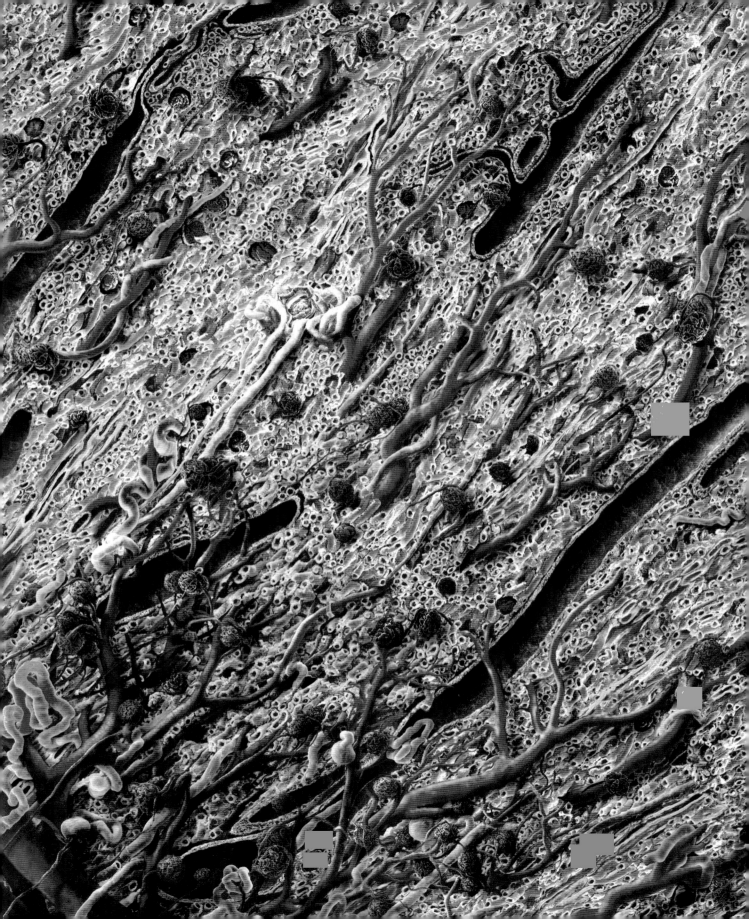

NEPHRON NETWORK

The kidneys are very densely packed organs comprised of winding and convoluted tubules and blood vessels that together create millions of tiny filtering units called nephrons.

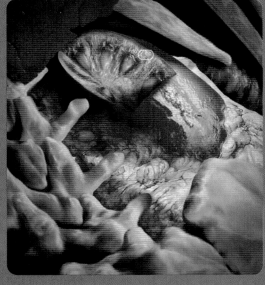

THERE ARE TWO TYPES OF NEPHRONS, BASED ON WHERE THEY ARE LOCATED IN THE KIDNEYS; CORTICAL NEPHRONS (HIGHLIGHTED) AND CORTICOMEDULLARY NEPHRONS (PORTION OF LATTER SHOWN IN LOWER LEFT CORNER).

INTO THE HEART OF THE KIDNEY

The nephron is composed of looping and folding tubules that at first glance look like an impossibly tangled knot of highways, side roads and interchanges. But in fact, the nephron directs the traffic flow effortlessly. When stretched out, a nephron would be almost a couple of feet in length and there are about a million nephrons in each kidney. A nephron is composed of two basic parts: the glomerulus and the tubule. The glomerulus, part of the vascular system, is a tuft of capillaries that filters the wastes and fluid from the blood. The tubules then catch, concentrate and excrete the waste into the urine.

The walls of the tubules are made of specialized cells, which serve as "check points" for the waste flowing by them. Hormonal sensors in these cells determine which substances should be excreted as waste and which substances will be reabsorbed into the blood to nourish the body's cells. The specific materials the cells are assigned to reabsorb or secrete include water and essential nutrients, salts and minerals, depending on where in the tubules the cells are located.

From the glomerulus until the collecting duct, intricate and minute calculations are at constant play within the nephron. The production of urine does not just result in a waste product but also protects the fine balance of substances required to keep the body healthy.

THE NEPHRON HAS SPECIALIZED AREAS WITH DIFFERENT FUNCTIONS.

1. Substances are filtered from blood plasma, except most proteins and blood cells.

2. Unnecessary substances are removed from the blood and secreted as filtrate.

3. Sixty-five percent of filtered water and sodium, plus small amounts of other substances, are reclaimed from tubular fluid and reabsorbed into the bloodstream.

4. Water moves according to a concentration gradient into or out of the vasa recta in order to concentrate the filtered waste.

5. Solutes such as sodium, chloride and urea are reabsorbed into the bloodstream.

6. Sodium, chloride, bicarbonate, potassium, calcium and magnesium are reabsorbed from the blood.

7. Communication between the macula densa of the distal tubules and the juxtaglomerular (JG) cells of the afferent arteriole helps the JG cells read and control blood pressure.

8. Sodium, chloride, bicarbonate, potassium and calcium are regulated.

9. The final product, urine, empties from the nephron into the collecting duct on its way out of the kidney to the bladder.

(4) DESCENDING LOOP OF HENLE

(5) ASCENDING LOOP OF HENLE

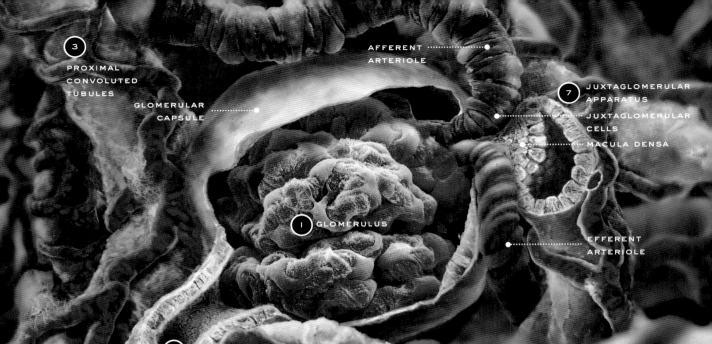

③ PROXIMAL
CONVOLUTED
TUBULES

GLOMERULAR
CAPSULE

AFFERENT
ARTERIOLE

⑦ JUXTAGLOMERULAR
APPARATUS

JUXTAGLOMERULAR
CELLS

MACULA DENSA

① GLOMERULUS

EFFERENT
ARTERIOLE

② PROXIMAL TUBULES

⑧ DISTAL
TUBULES

⑥ THICK ASCENDING LIMB
OF LOOP OF HENLE

CAPILLARY NETWORK
AROUND TUBULES
(VASA RECTA)

⑨ COLLECTIING
DUCT

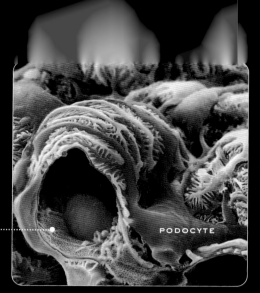

BASEMENT
MEMBRANE

PODOCYTE

VIEW OF A PODOCYTE WRAPPING AROUND
A FENESTRATED CAPILLARY

SMOOTH MUSCLE CELLS WRAP
AROUND AND CONSTRICT THE
AFFERENT ARTERIOLE HELPING
TO KEEP BLOOD PRESSURE
UNDER CONTROL.

AFFERENT ARTERIOLE

PROXIMAL
TUBULES

GLOMERULAR
CAPSULE

PODOCYTE

GLOMERULUS:
COMPOSED OF TIGHTLY
PACKED BLOOD VESSELS

EFFERENT
ARTERIOLE

CAPILLARY
NETWORK AROUND
DISTAL TUBULES

The glomerulus is the nephron's main filtering unit. The incoming renal artery enters the pelvis of the kidney, splits into four or five parts, and then ultimately branches into a dense thicket of interlobular arteries. These will each branch off into multiple glomeruli, tightly compact balls of capillaries that sit within membranes called Bowman's capsules.

The cells lining the inside of the glomerular capillaries are perforated with over a million tiny holes called fenestrations, making it possible for selective filtering of various wastes. Wrapped around these capillaries are specialized cells called podocytes. The layer of fenestrated capillaries and podocytes creates a semi-permeable filter through which water and soluble wastes can pass.

The kidneys also measure oxygen levels in the RBCs streaming through these capillaries. As soon as the kidneys detect below-normal oxygen levels in the blood, they release the hormone EPO into the bloodstream, sending it on its way to the bone marrow. It is EPO's job to then initiate RBC production in the marrow's stem cells. The production of EPO depends directly on the kidneys' ability to measure and detect changing oxygen levels. It is another example of the finely-tuned balancing act constantly being performed by our kidneys.

THE GLOMERULUS AND EPO AT WORK

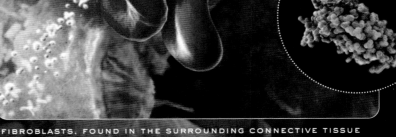

ENDOTHELIAL CELL

FIBROBLAST

THE EPO MOLECULE

DISTAL TUBULE

FIBROBLASTS, FOUND IN THE SURROUNDING CONNECTIVE TISSUE OF THE DISTAL TUBULES, AND ENDOTHELIAL CELLS OF CAPILLARIES ARE RESPONSIBLE FOR THE PRODUCTION OF EPO.

STEM/PROGENITOR CELL
STEM CELL COMES FROM THE LATIN *STEMME*, MEANING TREE TRUNK, AND *CELLA*, MEANING STOREROOM—A FITTING DESCRIPTION. THE STEM CELL IS A POWERHOUSE THAT STORES GENETIC INSTRUCTIONS (DNA) FOR CREATING RBCS AND OTHER TYPES OF CELLS AND IS READY TO SUPPLY THE BLOOD AND BODY WITH EVERY CELL NEEDED FOR HEALTHY FUNCTION.

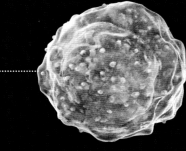

EPO ENTERS BONE MARROW THROUGH BLOOD VESSELS.

4 EPO IS IN THE BONE MARROW, SURROUNDED BY MILLIONS OF CELLS, INCLUDING STEM CELLS.

1 THE KIDNEY PRODUCES EPO.

3

2 EPO TRAVELS FROM THE KIDNEYS INTO BLOOD CIRCULATION.

EPO REACHES BONE MARROW.

2 IN SYNC: WHEN BLOOD AND THE KIDNEYS WORK TOGETHER

A RED BLOOD
CELL IS BORN

PO is produced by the kidney and travels through the
lood to the bones and into the marrow where it binds to
eceptors in the walls of stem cells. This union triggers a
eries of events inside the stem cells that instruct its DNA
o transform the cell into a RBC.

(5) EPO BINDS TO RECEPTORS ON THE SUR-
FACE OF A STEM/PROGENITOR CELL, ACTI-
VATING A CHAIN OF EVENTS WITHIN THAT
START THE STEM CELL'S MATURATION INTO
A RED BLOOD CELL.

EPO

EPO RECEPTOR

STEM CELL MEMBRANE

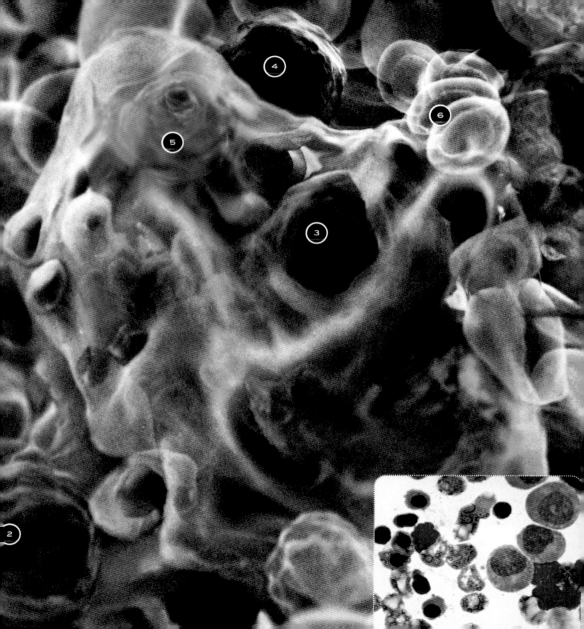

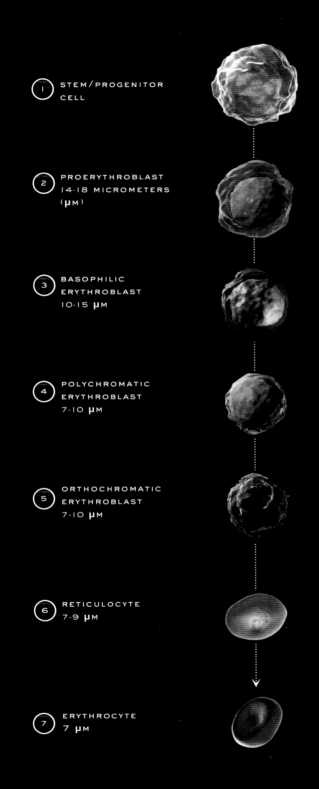

1. STEM/PROGENITOR CELL

2. PROERYTHROBLAST 14-18 MICROMETERS (μM)

3. BASOPHILIC ERYTHROBLAST 10-15 μM

4. POLYCHROMATIC ERYTHROBLAST 7-10 μM

5. ORTHOCHROMATIC ERYTHROBLAST 7-10 μM

6. RETICULOCYTE 7-9 μM

7. ERYTHROCYTE 7 μM

RBC PRODUCTION IN BONE MARROW

It is easy to think of bones only in terms of their structural function. But of course our bones are much more than scaffolding. Bone is biological tissue and the marrow is its living core. An average adult has less than six pounds of bone marrow, and yet that is responsible for producing all of the body's RBCs, platelets and most of the leukocytes found in the blood.

The interior bone marrow is soft, spongy and teeming with active cells. But even the hard exterior of bones is porous, which allows blood vessels to deliver EPO, the kidney's messenger molecule, to the marrow. These blood vessels, called sinuses, also provide direct routes by which the newly formed cells enter the bloodstream.

The production of the RBCs begins when EPO is transported by the blood to the bone marrow, where it binds to the stem cells. In the early stages of RBC development, the cells possess the "equipment" necessary for producing hemoglobin. Each cell has a nucleus, which holds the instructions for building the hemoglobin molecule; ribosomes, which have the manufacturing capacity to assemble the globin proteins; and mitochondria, which have the ability to synthesize the heme component.

This production capacity is short-lived, however. Before entering the bloodstream, the maturing RBC spits out its nucleus and all its internal organelles, which means that the mature RBC can no longer create the components of hemoglobin.

However, getting rid of its nucleus makes plenty of room for the millions of hemoglobin molecules inside the cell and provides for the cell's great flexibility. After about seven days, the cell is a fully mature erythrocyte, or RBC, equipped with its vital cargo of hemoglobin molecules, and is ready to enter the bloodstream. This critical process of blood cell production and delivery continues throughout a healthy person's lifetime.

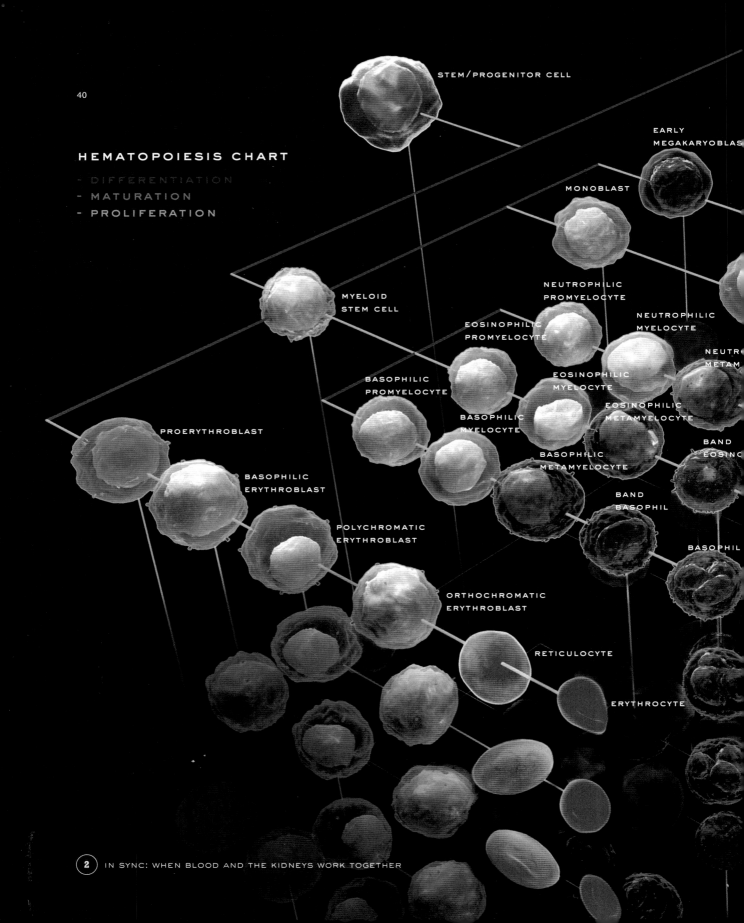

STEM/PROGENITOR CELL

EARLY
MEGAKARYOBLAST

MONOBLAST

HEMATOPOIESIS CHART
- DIFFERENTIATION
- MATURATION
- PROLIFERATION

NEUTROPHILIC
PROMYELOCYTE

MYELOID
STEM CELL

NEUTROPHILIC
MYELOCYTE

EOSINOPHILIC
PROMYELOCYTE

NEUTRO
METAM

BASOPHILIC
PROMYELOCYTE

EOSINOPHILIC
MYELOCYTE

EOSINOPHILIC
METAMYELOCYTE

PROERYTHROBLAST

BASOPHILIC
MYELOCYTE

BAND
EOSINO

BASOPHILIC
ERYTHROBLAST

BASOPHILIC
METAMYELOCYTE

BAND
BASOPHIL

POLYCHROMATIC
ERYTHROBLAST

BASOPHIL

ORTHOCHROMATIC
ERYTHROBLAST

RETICULOCYTE

ERYTHROCYTE

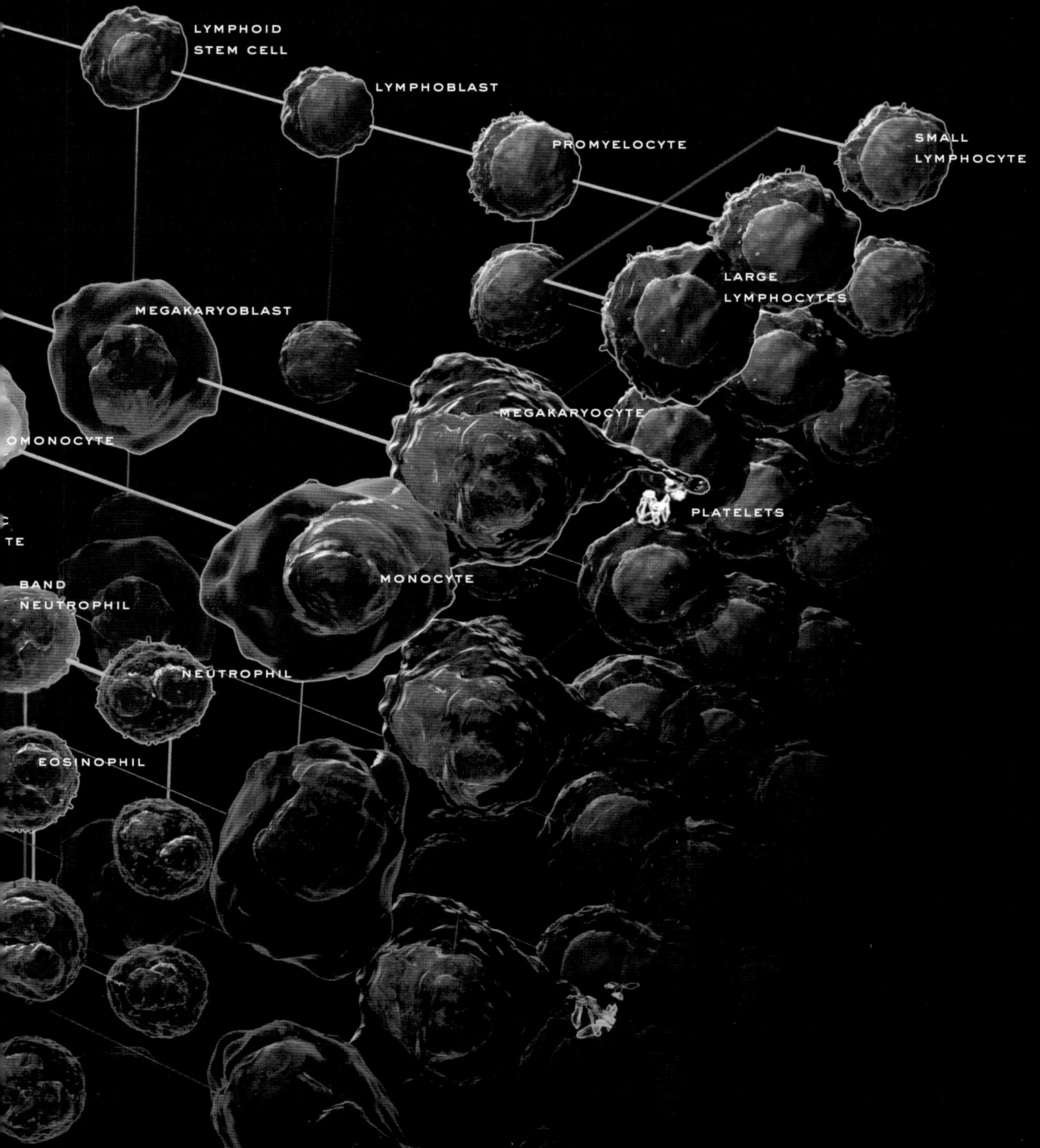

LYMPHOID
STEM CELL

LYMPHOBLAST

PROMYELOCYTE

SMALL
LYMPHOCYTE

LARGE
LYMPHOCYTES

MEGAKARYOBLAST

OMONOCYTE

MEGAKARYOCYTE

PLATELETS

TE

BAND
NEUTROPHIL

MONOCYTE

NEUTROPHIL

EOSINOPHIL

E UNUM PLURIBUS,
FROM ONE MANY

Many cells can result from one stem cell. Because division can occur at different stages of the cell's development, a single cell has the potential to become eight
to 32 RBCs.

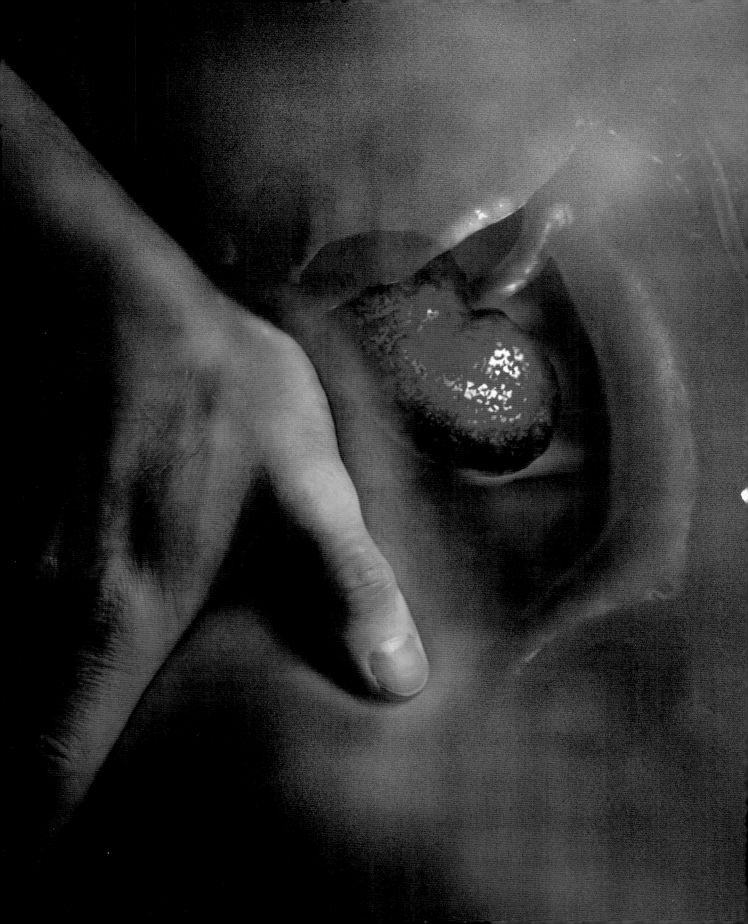

3

OFF BALANCE: WHEN THINGS GO WRONG

Chronic kidney disease (CKD) is the progressive, irreversible deterioration of kidney function. In this chapter, we will explain how CKD creates problems for the entire body and how it is intimately related to other diseases. You will learn how undetected and unmanaged diabetes and hypertension can damage your kidneys. And we will also explain the dangerous link between CKD and anemia and why anemia is not only a major complication of CKD, but also a contributor to CKD.

CKD: WHAT CAUSES IT AND WHY

Chronic kidney disease develops over time. It may occur because of an inherited susceptibility to kidney disease, such as cystic kidney disease, or as the result of other conditions such as diabetes or hypertension.

HYPERTENSION
Occurs when chronically high blood pressure is forced against blood vessel walls and damages the intricate vasculature of the kidney

DIABETES
Occurs when your body fails to produce and utilize insulin that is necessary in order to stabilize blood glucose (sugar) levels. High blood sugar causes damage to your kidneys and other organs

OBSTRUCTIONS IN THE URINARY TRACT
Caused by tumors, kidney stones or an enlarged prostate (in males)

CYSTIC KIDNEY DISEASE
An inherited disease which causes large cysts to form and expand in the kidneys, resulting in a loss of functional renal tubules

GLOMERULONEPHRITIS
A group of diseases that cause inflammation of the kidneys' glomeruli, which may be caused by a systemic disease such as a streptococcal infection

RECURRENT URINARY INFECTIONS

DEVELOPMENTAL MALFORMATIONS
Causes abnormal conditions of the urinary tract

AUTOIMMUNE DISEASES
Diseases, such as lupus, that cause the immune system to turn against the body and attack organs, including the kidney

VISUAL MANIFESTATIONS OF SOME COMMON CAUSES OF CKD

VASCULAR DAMAGE
DAMAGE DUE TO DISEASES SUCH AS HYPERTENSION AND DIABETES

OBSTRUCTIVE UROPATHY
OBSTRUCTION OF THE FLOW OF URINE FROM THE KIDNEYS ANYWHERE IN THE URINARY TRACT. FOR EXAMPLE, A CANCEROUS TUMOR OR A KIDNEY STONE WITHIN THE URETER OFTEN RESULTS IN IMPAIRMENT OF KIDNEY FUNCTION.

CYSTIC KIDNEY DISEASE
AN ABNORMAL CONDITION RESULTING OFTEN IN AN ENLARGED KIDNEY CONTAINING MANY CYSTS. MAY BE ACQUIRED, CONGENITAL OR INHERITED SUCH AS AUTOSOMAL DOMINANT POLYCYSTIC KIDNEY DISEASE.

GLOMERULONEPHRITIS
DAMAGE TO THE KIDNEYS CAUSED BY INFLAMMATION OF THE GLOMERULI

RECURRENT INFECTIONS

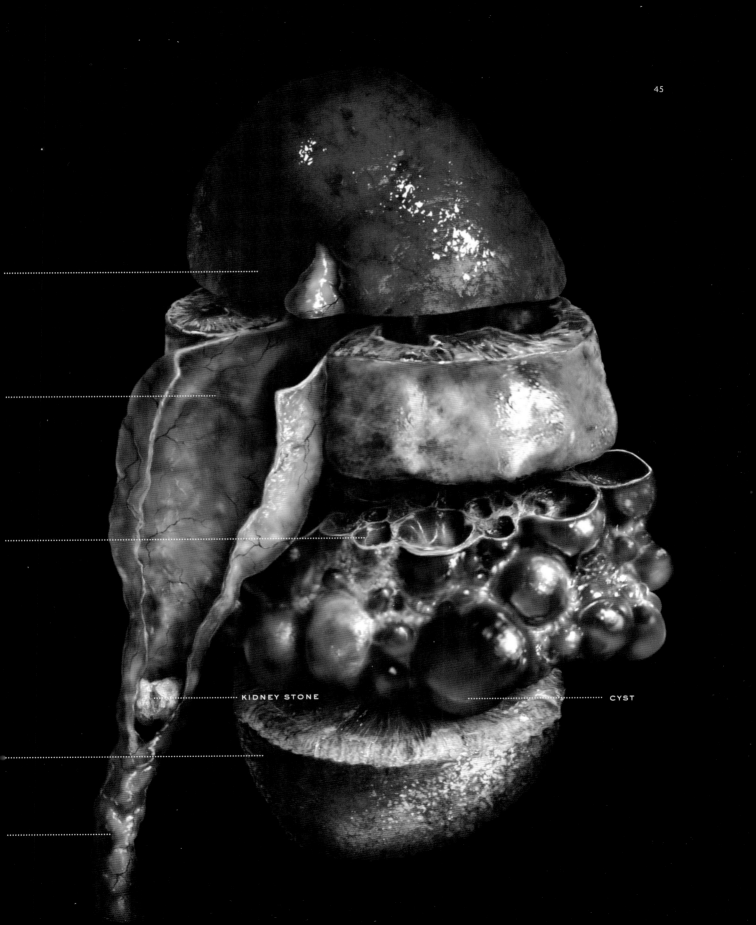

KIDNEY STONE

CYST

Hypertension is often referred to as the "silent killer," because it can cause no symptoms and go undetected for years. And as hypertension goes undiagnosed, the delicate linings of your blood vessels are being damaged, particularly those of the heart, the kidneys, and the eyes.

Hypertension is another word for high blood pressure; it has nothing to do with whether a person is considered tense or high-strung. Blood pressure is the measurement of the force the blood exerts as it pushes against the walls of your arteries. Your blood pres-sure is measured by a blood pressure cuff that is wrapped around your upper arm. Originally the read-ings referred to the height of a displaced column of mercury, but as in thermometers, the mercury yardstick is giving way to digital technologies. The "top" or first number—systolic pressure—represents the blood's pres-sure as the heart is contracted. The "bottom" or second number—diastolic pressure—represents the blood's pressure in the vessels when the heart is relaxed. Normal blood pressure is in the range of 120 (systolic) over 70 (diastolic).

HYPERTENSION: BLOOD PRESSURE'S DANGER ZONE

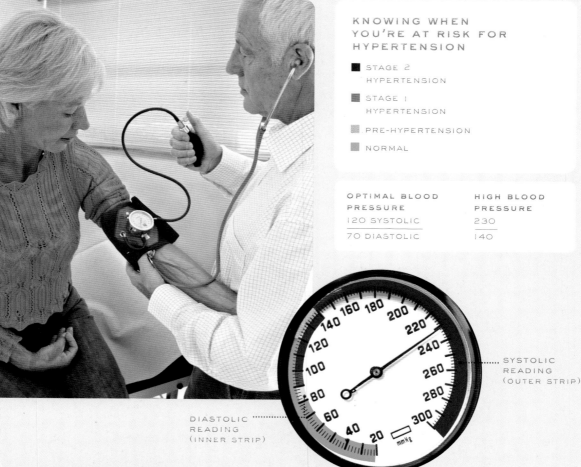

KNOWING WHEN YOU'RE AT RISK FOR HYPERTENSION

■ STAGE 2 HYPERTENSION

▨ STAGE 1 HYPERTENSION

▧ PRE-HYPERTENSION

▨ NORMAL

OPTIMAL BLOOD PRESSURE	HIGH BLOOD PRESSURE
120 SYSTOLIC	230
70 DIASTOLIC	140

DIASTOLIC READING (INNER STRIP)

SYSTOLIC READING (OUTER STRIP)

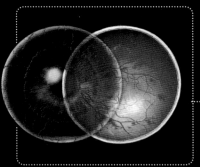

BLINDNESS

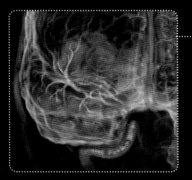

STROKE

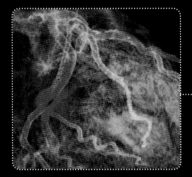

HEART ATTACK

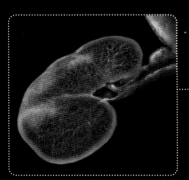

CHRONIC KIDNEY DISEASE

HOW HYPERTENSION CAN DAMAGE MULTIPLE BODY SYSTEMS

ALL YOUR ORGANS DEPEND ON BLOOD VESSELS TO FUNCTION. YOUR DELICATE ARTERIOLES AND CAPILLARIES, THE SMALLEST VESSELS, ARE INITIALLY DAMAGED WHEN HYPERTENSION OCCURS.

Hypertension can silently damage all of the blood vessels in your kidney, from the large renal artery to the tiny glomerular capillaries. Chronic high pressure on your artery walls causes them to expand, then break, scar and remodel, causing reduction in blood vessel diameter and further increasing blood pressure. Your arteries lose flexibility and are unable to contract and dilate in order to control blood flow. Smaller arteries, called arterioles, that enter and exit the glomerular tufts also become stiff and damaged. As hypertension progresses, the walls of your capillaries in your glomeruli may actually shrivel up, making it difficult for any blood cells to pass through.

Your kidneys are extremely vulnerable to hypertension because kidneys are "end organs," which means that they contain terminal or "end arteries." There is a single main artery, the renal artery, that supplies blood to the kidneys. This main artery, in turn, branches into smaller and smaller vessels. But among these smaller branches there are very few interconnections. So if the renal artery is damaged, the smaller vessels that branch from this renal artery are also affected. And because there is no other main arterial source of blood, the result is that there is no alternate route that can help to supply the vessels and tissues downstream with nutrients and oxygen. The areas of your kidney that are deprived of an adequate blood supply can no longer function and will die. When hypertension is severe enough, kidney damage becomes permanent, and eventually CKD may occur. The worse the hypertension, the more likely CKD will result.

HOW HYPERTENSION HARMS YOUR KIDNEYS

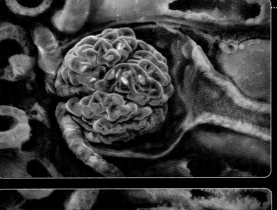

NORMAL GLOMERULUS
BLOOD FLOWS EASILY THROUGH (SUFFICIENTLY) WIDE GLOMERULAR CAPILLARIES.

HYPERTENSIVE GLOMERULUS
BASEMENT MEMBRANE OF THE GLOMERULAR CAPSULE THICKENS. CONNECTIVE TISSUE OVERTAKES THE NORMAL TISSUE THAT SURROUNDS THE HEALTHY GLOMERULUS. EVENTUALLY THE GLOMERULAR CAPILLARIES SHRINK AND HARDEN LEAVING THE GLOMERULUS UNABLE TO FUNCTION.

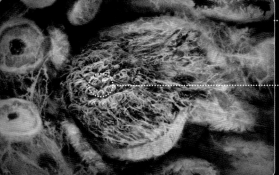

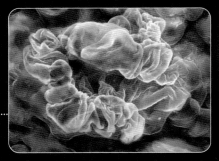

HYPERTENSIVE GLOMERULAR CAPILLARIES DEVELOP WRINKLES THAT OBSTRUCT THE OPEN SPACE WITHIN THE VESSEL, OR LUMEN, AND IMPEDE BLOOD FLOW.

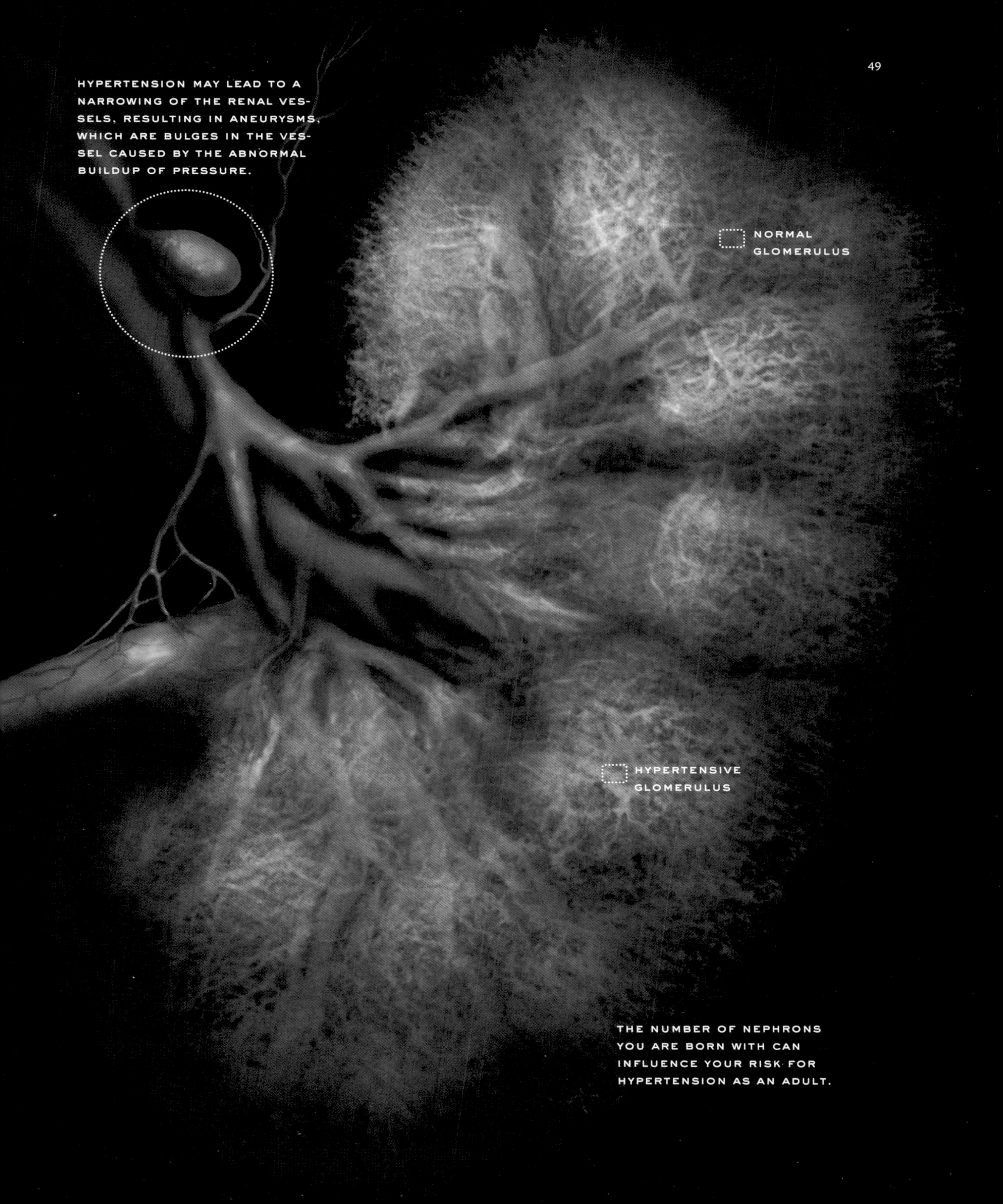

HYPERTENSION MAY LEAD TO A NARROWING OF THE RENAL VES-SELS, RESULTING IN ANEURYSMS, WHICH ARE BULGES IN THE VES-SEL CAUSED BY THE ABNORMAL BUILDUP OF PRESSURE.

NORMAL GLOMERULUS

HYPERTENSIVE GLOMERULUS

THE NUMBER OF NEPHRONS YOU ARE BORN WITH CAN INFLUENCE YOUR RISK FOR HYPERTENSION AS AN ADULT.

Diabetes is the number one cause of CKD and is responsible for 60 percent of the cases of CKD that eventually result in kidney failure. One hundred eighty million people worldwide suffer from diabetes, and many of them don't even know it—at least not yet. This means that approximately 5.1 percent of the world's population suffers from the disease and its consequences. People with diabetes cannot break down glucose in their blood because they can't produce or properly use a hormone called insulin that keeps blood glucose levels normal. Insulin is essential for converting food into energy.

Diabetes initially affects the smaller blood vessels in your body such as capillaries; this is because too much glucose can break down these delicate capillary walls. As a consequence symptoms occur first in tissues and organs whose function relies on an extensive capillary network, such as your kidneys and eyes, and in extremities, such as fingers and toes.

DIABETES: UPSETTING BLOOD'S BALANCE

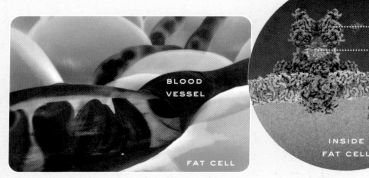

FAT AND MUSCLE CELLS UTILIZE GLUCOSE (PINK) AVOIDING GLUCOSE BUILD UP IN THE BLOODSTREAM.

NORMAL INSULIN FUNCTION

INSULIN RECEPTOR
INSULIN
GLUCOSE ENTERING A CELL

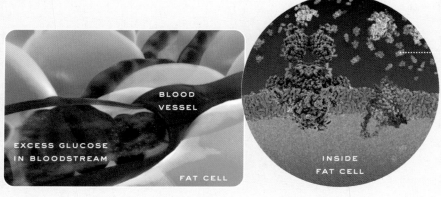

IN A DIABETIC PERSON, INSULIN IS EITHER NOT PRODUCED OR NOT ABLE TO BE UTILIZED PROPERLY, LEADING TO AN ABNORMAL BUILD-UP OF GLUCOSE (PINK) IN THE BLOODSTREAM.

TYPE II DIABETES

GLUCOSE IN THE BLOODSTREAM

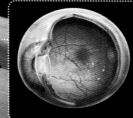

DIABETIC RETINOPATHY (RETINAL BLOOD VESSEL DAMAGE OF THE EYE)

NUMEROUS YELLOW PATCHES ARE SEEN ON THE MACULA AT THE BACK OF THE EYEBALL. THESE ARE EXUDATES THAT HAVE LEAKED FROM THE PERMEABLE BLOOD VESSELS IN CASES OF UNCONTROLLED DIABETES, CAUSING IRREVERSIBLE VISION LOSS.

COMMON COMPLICATIONS OF DIABETES
- ERECTILE DYSFUNCTION
- NEUROPATHIES (NERVE DAMAGE) OF THE EYE, STOMACH, AND PERIPHERAL NERVOUS SYSTEM
- KIDNEY DISEASE

PANCREAS:
SITE OF INSULIN
PRODUCTION

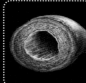

ERECTILE DYSFUNCTION

PERIPHERAL BLOOD VESSELS BECOME DAMAGED IN UNCONTROLLED DIABETES, MAKING IT IMPOSSIBLE FOR THE PENIS TO BECOME ENGORGED WITH BLOOD AND ERECT.

GANGRENE

PERIPHERAL NERVE DAMAGE RESULTS IN LOSS OF SENSATION, WHICH INCREASES THE RISK OF INJURY AND GANGRENE (TISSUE DEATH).

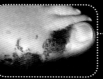

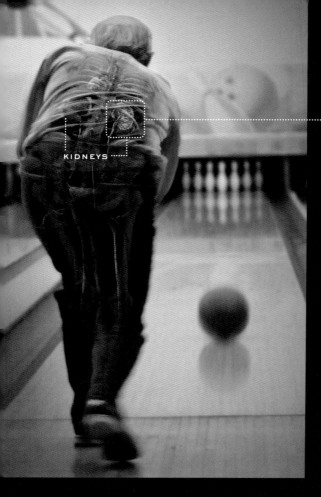

KIDNEYS

NEPHRON

GLOMERULUS

HOW DIABETES DAMAGES YOUR KIDNEYS

Diabetes and CKD are intimately related. In fact a third of all patients who will be diagnosed with diabetes will also develop CKD. When blood glucose levels are out of control, the kidneys become overtaxed and they cannot process the excessive amounts of glucose that should be removed from the blood.

Diabetes initially affects the smallest vessels in your body, the capillaries, and these capillaries are essential to the key functioning unit of your kidneys, the nephron. Indeed millions of capillaries, along with

specialized cells called podocytes, help to form the filter in the glomerulus. So when diabetes breaks down the kidney capillaries, it is destroying the kidney's main filtration units. Proteins in the blood's liquid plasma that should stay in the bloodstream instead leak across the diseased capillary wall into the waste stream. Doctors can diagnose kidney damage by measuring excess levels of protein in a patient's urine, a condition called proteinuria.

CROSS-SECTION OF THE THREE-LAYER
FILTRATION MEMBRANE COMPOSED OF CAPILLARY
ENDOTHELIUM, BASEMENT MEMBRANE, AND
PODOCYTE FOOT PROCESSES. SMALL PROTEINS
(GREEN) SOMETIMES LEAK THROUGH THESE
LAYERS OF THE DAMAGED CAPILLARIES.

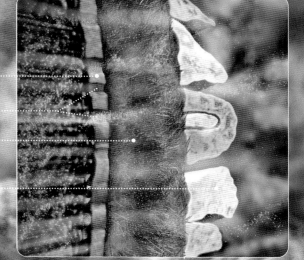

CAPILLARY
ENDOTHELIUM

FENESTRATIONS IN
ENDOTHELIUM

BASEMENT
MEMBRANE

PODOCYTE FOOT
PROCESS (PEDICLE)

CROSS-SECTION OF THE
GLOMERULAR CAPILLARY

DOMINO EFFECT: CKD, ANEMIA AND EPO

The kidneys are the site of EPO production. The hormone EPO is critical to our overall vitality because it stimulates the production of new RBCs, which contain hemoglobin—the oxygen dispenser for all the body's cells. When kidney function deteriorates, the production of EPO is compromised and fewer RBCs are created.

The chain reaction goes like this: Once the kidneys are damaged, less EPO is dispatched to the marrow, and RBC production declines. This means there is less hemoglobin available and the body's cells, including kidney cells, receive less oxygen. With less oxygen kidney function declines further, which means even less EPO production and even lower RBC levels. The result is anemia—illustrating why anemia goes hand-in-hand with CKD.

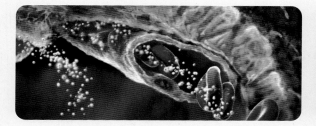

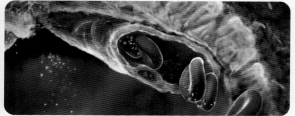

HEALTHY

THE KIDNEYS PRODUCE EPO IN RESPONSE TO LOW OXYGEN LEVELS IN ORDER TO STIMULATE RED BLOOD CELL PRODUCTION IN THE BONE MARROW. A NORMAL AMOUNT OF RED BLOOD CELLS ALLOWS FOR THE DELIVERY OF AN ADEQUATE SUPPLY OF OXYGEN.

UNHEALTHY

IN CKD THE EPO-PRODUCING CELLS ARE UNABLE TO FUNCTION PROPERLY SO THERE IS LESS EPO REACHING THE BONE MARROW. LOWER EPO LEVELS IN THE BONE MARROW CAUSE DECREASED RED BLOOD CELL PRODUCTION. FEWER RED BLOOD CELLS LEAD TO A LACK OF OXYGEN AND EVENTUALLY ANEMIA.

When Kent was suffering from CKD and anemia, he was constantly tired. "If [I] had time to sleep that's what [I was] doing: I was sleeping," Kent recalled.

A VICIOUS CYCLE: CKD, ANEMIA AND HEART DISEASE

Hypertension, diabetes, obesity, cardiovascular disease, CKD and anemia have much in common. In fact it can be difficult to determine where, exactly, one ends and another begins. Sometimes one disease can be both a cause and consequence of another disease. But the good news is that if you do something to decrease the risk factors for one disease, you decrease your risk for the others as well.

Millions of people worldwide suffer from anemia. All anemias, not just anemia associated with CKD, can have an impact on other medical conditions. Anemia can affect the ability of the heart to function and, thereby, increase the risk of heart disease and cardiovascular failure. Once anemia accompanies heart disease in a patient, things only get worse for the already overworked heart. When the blood is depleted of oxygen, the heart must work harder to pump more blood to try to meet the increased need. If the anemia becomes chronic, the heart is even more overworked, and this can throw the heart's normal electrical rhythm off balance, which can in turn lead to a heart attack. Without medical intervention, the cycle continues, and permanent damage occurs.

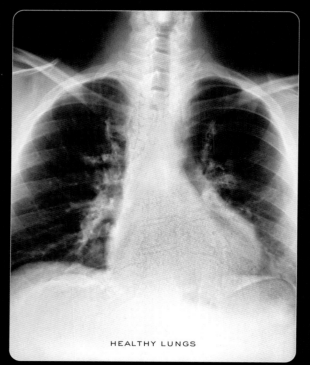

HEALTHY LUNGS

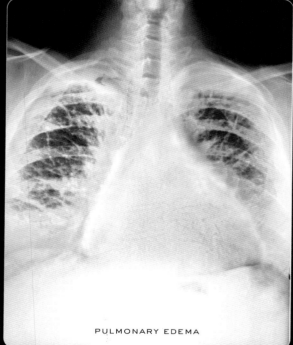

PULMONARY EDEMA

WHEN THE HEART IS PUMPING PLENTY OF BLOOD, OXYGEN IS ABLE TO REACH ALL OF THE BODY'S TISSUES.

WHEN THE HEART NO LONGER PUMPS ADEQUATE AMOUNTS OF BLOOD TO THE BODY'S TISSUES, FLUID WASTE BEGINS TO BACK UP INTO THE LUNGS, MAKING IT DIFFICULT TO BREATHE.

SEVERE ANEMIA

IN ANEMIA, OXYGEN DELIVERY TO THE BODY'S TISSUES IS COMPROMISED. THE HEART DOES ITS BEST TO COMPENSATE BY PUMPING HARDER. BECAUSE OF THE EXTRA WORK, THE HEART MUSCLE ENLARGES, LEADING TO DAMAGE.

ENLARGED HEART AND CONGESTIVE HEART FAILURE

CHRONIC KIDNEY DISEASE

WHEN THE KIDNEYS ARE DAMAGED, THEY DON'T PRODUCE ENOUGH EPO FOR ADEQUATE RED BLOOD CELL PRODUCTION. THIS LACK OF RED BLOOD CELLS EXACERBATES ANEMIA, MAKING THE HEART PUMP EVEN HARDER AND CAUSING MORE DAMAGE.

OTHER CONDITIONS THAT ARE CONNECTED TO CKD AND ANEMIA

Chronic anemia can seriously affect a whole spectrum of other disorders.

BONE DISEASE

The most common bone disorder associated with CKD is when bone is unable to metabolize key elements such as phosphorous and calcium. The consequence is that bones can weaken, become painful and may eventually break.

EXERCISE FUNCTION

Anemia can limit a person's ability to exercise and reduce the body's endurance in general. The result can be that a person is forced to stop in mid-stride due to lack of breath, dizziness and feeling faint.

SLEEP DISTURBANCES

Some people who suffer from chronic anemia develop sleep problems, possibly because their bodies are not getting enough oxygen.

RISK OF CANCER

The presence of anemia, especially in the elderly, may be a predictor of an increased risk for cancer compared to elderly people without anemia.

If you have chronic anemia, no matter what the original cause, you should discuss treatment options with your doctor. These might include synthetic EPO treatment. Controlling chronic anemia can improve overall health and quality of life as well as prevent or improve other medical conditions.

RESULTS OF MAGNETIC RESONANCE IMAGING (MRI)

A HEALTHY OLDER BRAIN
IN THE BRAIN OF A PERSON WHO IS AGING WELL, ADEQUATE AMOUNTS OF BLOOD REACH THE BRAIN TO SUPPLY IT WITH OXYGEN.

BRAIN WITH VASCULAR DEMENTIA
WHEN BLOOD VESSELS ARE DAMAGED, THE BRAIN DOES NOT RECEIVE ENOUGH OXYGEN. THIS CAN LEAD TO EARLY ONSET DEMENTIA.

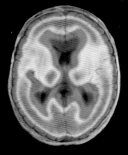

REGIONS WITH HIGH BLOOD FLOW ARE DISPLAYED AS ORANGE TO WHITE. REGIONS WITH LOWER BLOOD FLOW ARE DISPLAYED AS BLUE TO BLACK.

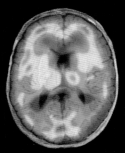

DEMENTIA

When the flow of oxygen to the brain is inhibited, brain tissue is damaged and function deteriorates. Chronic anemia is being studied now in terms of its effects on cognitive retention. Studies have confirmed the connection between anemia and signs of dementia in people over 65.

CELLS THAT DIVIDE QUICKLY IN THE BODY

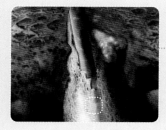

HAIR ROOT
IN SKIN

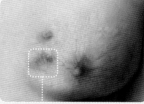

CELLS DIVIDING
IN HAIR FOLLICLE

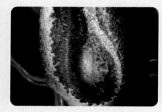

TUMOR WITHIN
BREAST TISSUE

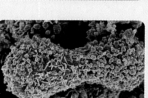

A CANCER CELL
DIVIDING

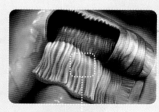

INTESTINAL WALL

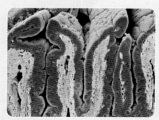

DIVIDING CELLS
WITHIN THE
INTESTINAL WALL

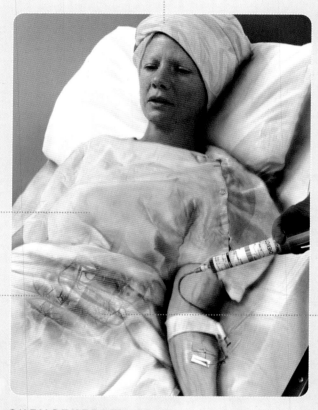

CHEMOTHERAPY

Chemotherapy kills the quickly dividing cells within the cancer tumor, inhibiting cell replication. But it also wreaks havoc with other rapidly dividing cells, such as the cells of the blood, gastrointestinal (GI) tract, and the hair follicles, resulting in anemia, nausea, diarrhea and hair loss, respectively.

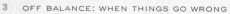

CANCER TREATMENT AND ANEMIA

In a few cases anemia may be caused by cancer itself. But in the majority of cases anemia results from the treatment, chemotherapy, because chemo kills all quickly dividing cells, like the stem cells that produce RBCs. Treatment of anemia with synthetic EPO can be very effective during the course of chemotherapy. When chemotherapy is completed, the patient is monitored to determine healthy RBC and hemoglobin levels before EPO injections can end.

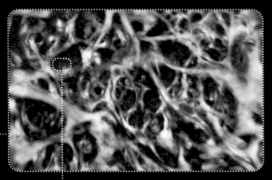

BONE MARROW

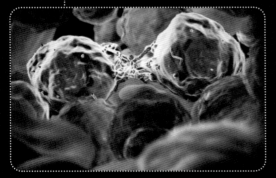

MATURING RED BLOOD CELL DIVIDING

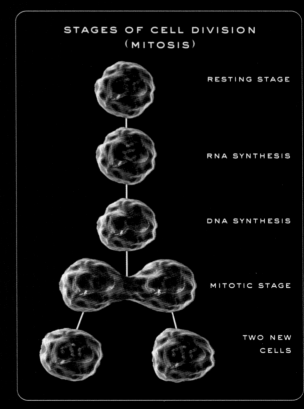

STAGES OF CELL DIVISION (MITOSIS)

RESTING STAGE

RNA SYNTHESIS

DNA SYNTHESIS

MITOTIC STAGE

TWO NEW CELLS

CHEMOTHERAPY KILLS ALL QUICKLY DIVIDING CELLS—NOT ONLY CANCER CELLS, BUT ALSO YOUR HEALTHY CELLS. CELLS ARE SUSCEPTIBLE DURING SPECIFIC STAGES (RED) OF DIVISION.

OTHER ANEMIAS: COMPROMISING THE BLOOD IN MANY WAYS

There are many other forms of anemia that affect overall health, some of which can be permanently damaging. Common anemias include sickle cell anemia, thalassemia and aplastic anemia. No matter what the cause is, if the anemia is not caught early and managed efficiently, kidney function can eventually be impaired. In serious cases of anemia, the loss of kidney function can be progressive. Pregnancy-related anemia is also common, but less dangerous.

APLASTIC ANEMIA
Aplastic anemia is a "one of a kind" anemia and is a very serious, life-threatening disease. It is, in fact, a bone marrow disorder rather than a blood disorder. In aplastic anemia, the stem cells in the bone marrow cease to function adequately and a dramatic decrease in the production of all blood cells occurs. It is usually caused by injury or abnormal suppression of the marrow itself. At present, the treatment with greatest success is bone marrow transplant.

THALASSEMIA
Thalassemia is an inherited disorder that results in low production of hemoglobin. The anemia associated with thalassemia could be severe and is accompanied by ineffective erythropoiesis. Thalassemia is a recessive trait; therefore it is carried by only one gene. If a child is born to parents who each carry this recessive trait, two serious situations may occur: 1) alpha-thalassemia, in which the hemoglobin lacks enough of the alpha-globin protein, or 2) beta-thalassemia or Cooley's anemia, which involves a lack of the beta-globin protein. Management for thalassemia usually involves transfusion therapy with accompanying hormone therapy. Thalassemia may be cured by bone marrow transplantation.

PREGNANCY-RELATED ANEMIA
In pregnancy-related anemia, the expectant mother's body is working double-time to provide oxygen to herself and to the fetus fed by the blood-rich, oxygen-rich placenta. It is easy to see how the necessity for additional iron atoms to bind oxygen may cause a drain on the system. Small doses of iron usually take care of pregnancy-related anemia without any difficulties.

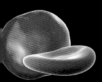

HEALTHY RED BLOOD CELLS

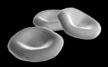

SMALLER RED BLOOD CELLS (THALASSEMIA)

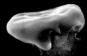

DYING (APOPTOSIS) RED BLOOD CELL

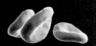

IRON DEFICIENT RED BLOOD CELLS RESULTING IN A LOSS OF RED COLOR (PREGNANCY-RELATED)

SICKLE CELL ANEMIA

Sickle cell anemia is also an inherited blood disorder. Like thalassemia, it is in a group of diseases caused by abnormal hemoglobin molecules. In sickle cell disease, the abnormal hemoglobin molecules stick to each other. This causes the RBCs to assume a crescent-like shape (which gives the disease its name) and the cells' surfaces to become rigid, the combination of which can cause the cells to become stuck in blood vessels. The disease also results in the early death of RBCs, sometimes after only a few weeks, compared to the usual 16 weeks. Sickle cell anemia commonly affects those with ancestors from Africa, the Middle East, the Mediterranean, or India. The treatment focuses on controlling the symptoms as long as possible. Blood transfusions are also used, and recent studies have shown that bone marrow transplants may offer hope, particularly in young children with severe cases. Still, early diagnosis is critical in managing sickle cell anemia.

CRISIS RESULTING IN ORGAN DAMAGE FROM SICKLING

CONGESTION OF CAPILLARY LOOPS IS EVIDENT IN THIS CASE OF SICKLE CELL CRISIS, WITH OCCASIONAL SICKLED RED BLOOD CELLS DISCERNIBLE (RIGHT).

SICKLE CELLS

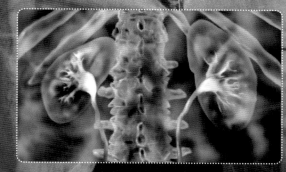

HOOKS (DAMAGED CALYCES)

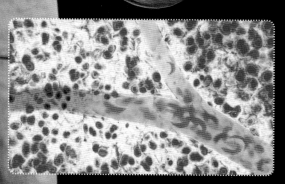

SICKLE CELL CRISIS

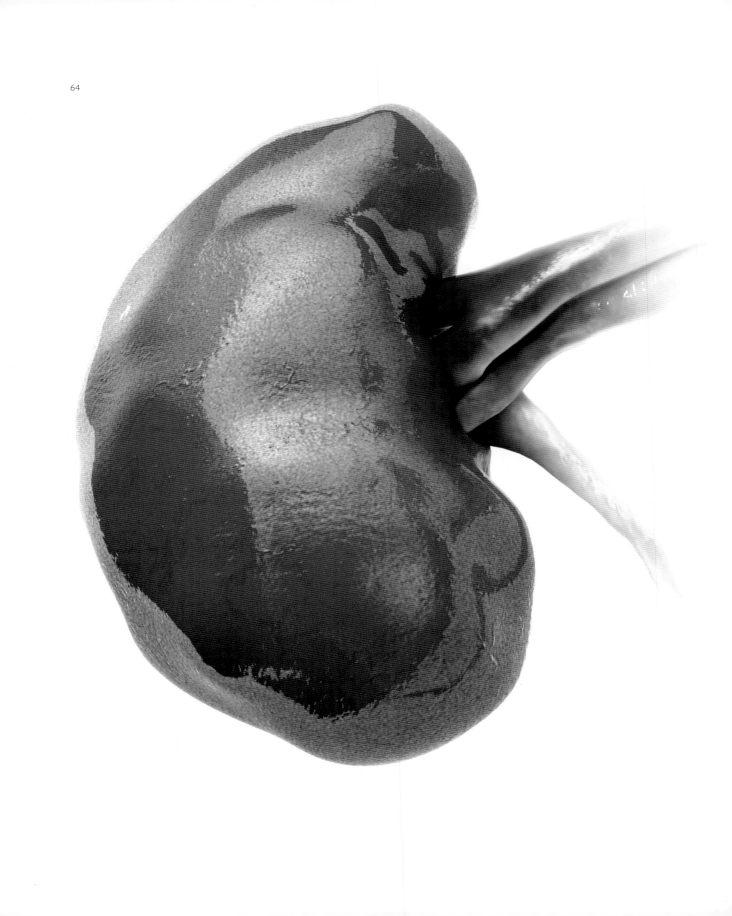

RECLAIMING BALANCE: DIAGNOSIS AND TREATMENT

Diagnosing CKD and related conditions is challenging because symptoms often don't appear until the disease has progressed and permanent kidney damage has already occurred. This is why it is essential that you understand the risk factors for CKD. You may be at risk for CKD if you have hypertension, diabetes, have a family history of the disease, belong to a population group that has high rates of hypertension or diabetes, such as African-American, Native American, Afro-Caribbean, Asian or Aboriginal people, or you are older than 65.

If you are at increased risk, it is important that you ask your primary care physician to screen you for CKD. If you show signs of CKD, the sooner you get started on finding your best treatment plan and implementing it, the more successful your treatment will be. While a diagnosis of CKD is never good news, taking positive action is the best way to deal with understandable feelings of anxiety and a sense of feeling overwhelmed.

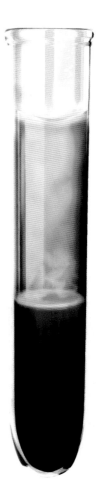

LIVING WITH KIDNEY DISEASE

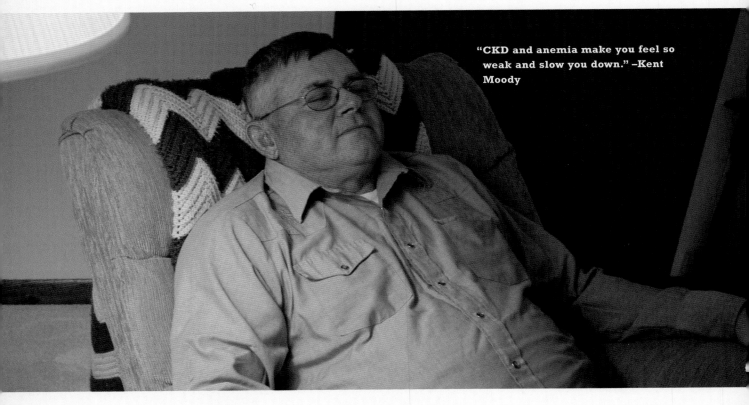

"CKD and anemia make you feel so weak and slow you down." –Kent Moody

Life on a farm is never easy, but for Kent Moody it's become nearly impossible. A fourth generation farmer, the 56 year-old from Crisman, Illinois, has been battling diabetes and high blood pressure for over 25 years, and the quarter of a century struggle has finally pushed his kidneys to near failure. No longer able to filter blood and water from his cells properly, Moody's kidneys are barely keeping him alive. "I just can't seem to get going," he says. "I'm just tired all the time. And I want to have a lifestyle where I'm not tired all the time so I can feel like being with people and family and seeing my grandkids."

Moody shares responsibility for 13,000 acres of crops with his brother and nephew. On most days they labor for 12 long hours operating tractors and combines; during planting and harvest season those days often stretch out to 18 hours. For Moody that pace is nearly impossible to maintain any longer. "When I sit in the tractor I can tell my legs start filling up with fluid," he says. "And I am so weak I can hardly pull myself up in a semi-tractor; I'm just so physically exhausted from one end to the other."

His doctors at Indiana University tell him that the

relentless strain produced by his hypertension have pushed his kidneys to their breaking point. To give his body some extra help, he takes 20 separate medications— 13 pills in the morning and 7 before going to bed to regulate his blood pressure and sugar levels. As a diabetic, Moody also wears an insulin pump, which he fills with the life-saving insulin his body can no longer provide but still needs in order to function. But the medications are not enough; they cannot make up for everything that his kidneys are supposed to do but can't. Every month Moody has a blood test to monitor his red blood cell count, and every month the number drops a little more. "I thought I could rest enough on the weekends to get going, but I can't, because my red blood cells were not repairing and rebuilding enough," he says. "I sleep every night in the chair for two or three hours before I go to bed." His dropping red cell count also makes Moody anemic, which means his muscles are not getting the iron they need to work properly, and causes his body temperature to drop.

Moody's exhaustion, however, is only physical. Mentally, he is as vital as he was before his kidneys began to fail. "I don't want to retire right now; I'm ready to go back to work and continue farming for a few more years," he says. As a grandfather, Moody wants to have enough energy to play ball and fish with his grandsons. "When you just sit down and quit that doesn't give you anything to do or look forward to or plan for. I've been busy all my life and I wouldn't want to sit around with not much to do."

So to give him some help, Moody's doctors have prescribed shots of EPO, a synthetic form of the naturally occurring erythropoietin normally produced by the kidneys. Erythropoietin stimulates the production of red blood cells, which carry much-needed oxygen and iron to tissues. Moody now gets an EPO shot once every three weeks to keep his red blood cell counts up. "We call it the Superman shot. Now I have so much more energy," he says.

But the shots are not a permanent solution. Moody's doctors have recommended that he have a kidney transplant, replacing his ailing organs with healthier ones that can bring his body back into balance and restore the energy that Moody so desperately needs. But before he can even be considered as a recipient for a donated kidney, he needs to register his blood type and ensure that he is medically qualified to receive a new kidney. He and his wife and daughter travel to Indiana University for a battery of tests. "They check about everything they can possibly check," he says. "They do a colonoscopy. I can't have any cancer in my body at all or they will throw us out. I had a heart test and they put me on a table and ran dye through me and did several other tests too."

Moody learns that he can become a recipient, but well-matched, donated kidneys are difficult to obtain. Making matters more challenging, he has type B negative blood, a rare combination. "They said you could be on a list and that [it will take] probably four to five years," he says. All he can do now is wait.

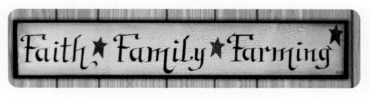

VALUES BY WHICH THE MOODYS LIVE

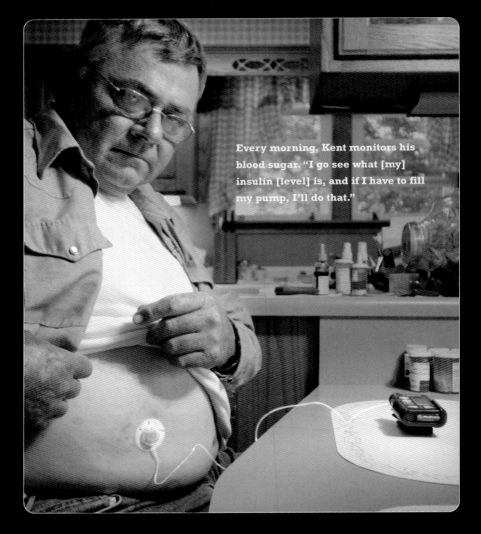

Every morning, Kent monitors his blood sugar. "I go see what [my] insulin [level] is, and if I have to fill my pump, I'll do that."

YOU AND YOUR GLUCOMETER

THE KEY TO THE MANAGEMENT OF DIABETES IS A DEVICE CALLED A GLUCOMETER. FROM A SINGLE DROP OF BLOOD PRODUCED BY A PIN PRICK, THE GLUCOMETER READS HOW MUCH SUGAR IS IN YOUR BLOOD. THE NORMAL RANGE IS 70-120 MG/DL. YOU SHOULD WRITE YOUR NUMBERS DOWN EVERY TIME, INCLUDING THE DAY AND TIME WHEN YOU TOOK THE TEST. AND SHARE THESE NUMBERS WITH YOUR HEALTH CARE TEAM.

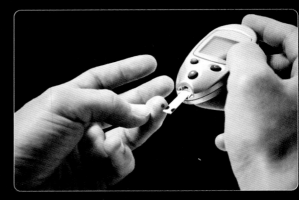

THE KEY TO SUCCESS: CONTROLLING DIABETES IN CKD

High blood sugar levels, which occur when diabetes goes uncontrolled, tax the kidneys as they try to remove all of the excess sugar as waste. Over time the kidneys' tiny blood vessels are damaged from the burden. While 30 percent of those with Type 1 diabetes and 40 percent of those with Type 2 diabetes may develop CKD, this does not have to happen. In Type 1 diabetes the body produces no insulin; in Type 2 diabetes, the most common, the body produces too little or can't use what it does produce. If you maintain your blood sugar levels within the normal range, you reduce your risk of kidney damage. If you have already been diagnosed with CKD, the sooner you begin to keep tight control over your blood sugar levels, the sooner you can put the brakes on further kidney damage.

Tight control can only occur if you limit sugar consumption and simple carbohydrate consumption, maintain a healthy weight, and increase exercise and overall physical activity. Diabetics who already have permanent kidney damage should limit the amount of protein in their diet, since a protein-rich diet can place additional stress on weakened kidneys.

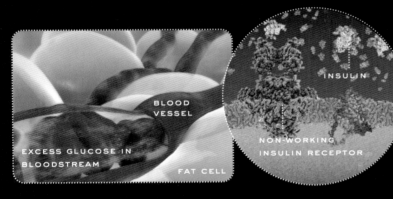

BLOOD VESSEL

INSULIN

NON-WORKING INSULIN RECEPTOR

EXCESS GLUCOSE IN BLOODSTREAM

FAT CELL

A DIABETIC'S ABNORMAL LEVEL OF GLUCOSE IN THE BLOODSTREAM
BECAUSE AVAILABLE INSULIN IS UNABLE TO BIND CORRECTLY TO THE INSULIN RECEPTOR, THE GLUCOSE CHANNELS DO NOT ALLOW GLUCOSE (PINK) TO MOVE FROM THE BLOODSTREAM TO THE WAITING CELLS.

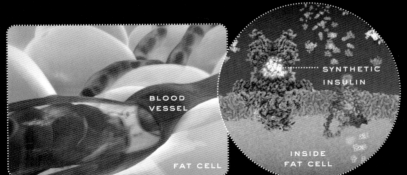

BLOOD VESSEL

SYNTHETIC INSULIN

FAT CELL

INSIDE FAT CELL

NORMALIZED BLOOD SUGAR AFTER MEDICATION
SYNTHETIC INSULIN MAKES IT POSSIBLE FOR THE IMPAIRED INSULIN RECEPTOR TO BEGIN TO WORK AGAIN AND THUS OPENS THE CHANNELS SO THAT GLUCOSE (PINK) MOVES FROM THE BLOOD TO CELLS.

STAYING AHEAD OF CKD: CONTROLLING HYPTERTENSION

Hypertension (high blood pressure) is a leading cause of CKD, second only to uncontrolled diabetes. Hypertension forces the heart to pump harder in order to deliver oxygen to the body's cells and remove waste through the blood and kidneys. Despite its hard work, the heart becomes less efficient. Eventually hypertension damages small blood vessels, including the kidney's vital filtering mechanisms, the nephrons.

Luckily there are many good ways to manage hypertension. First, if you smoke, you must stop. Smoking causes your blood vessels to constrict, which in turn can lead to hypertension, since the blood is being forced through narrower channels. If you are overweight, shedding excess pounds will help ease the burden on the heart muscle. Above all else, increasing the amount of exercise you get every day will also strengthen the heart.

If you are unable to control your hypertension on your own, your doctor may prescribe medication, such as ACE inhibitors, to help lower blood pressure. ACE inhibitors work by inhibiting the action of a natural enzyme, angiotensin, that causes blood vessel constriction.

CONDITIONS ASSOCIATED WITH HYPERTENSION

OBESITY: Approximately 1.6 billion adults are overweight and at least 400 million are obese worldwide. By 2015 it is projected that these numbers will increase to 2.3 billion overweight and more than 700,000 obese adults. Obesity raises the risk of disease across the board and is a primary cause of hypertension.

CIGARETTE SMOKING: Smoking cigarettes can damage your overall health. In addition to causing your blood vessels to constrict, smoking puts you at greater risk for heart and lung disease as well as kidney and bladder cancer. Many of the carcinogens (cancer-causing substances) from smoking are absorbed through the lungs into the bloodstream and then filtered through the kidneys, where they can damage cells before going to the bladder to be excreted as urine.

PHYSICAL INACTIVITY: If you are not physically active, you have at least a 35 percent higher risk of hypertension.

EXCESSIVE ALCOHOL CONSUMPTION: Consuming large quantities of alcohol affects your overall health and can put you at risk for high blood pressure. Although it is proven that consuming alcohol causes blood pressure to increase, it isn't clear exactly how this happens. Alcohol may cause blood pressure-elevating hormones to be overproduced, or alter the balance of electrolytes (sodium, potassium, magnesium and calcium), which in turn causes capillaries to constrict and blood pressure to increase.

KENT MOODY DOES NOT DRINK OR SMOKE, BUT ABUSE OF ALCOHOL AND TOBACCO CAN RESULT IN CKD.

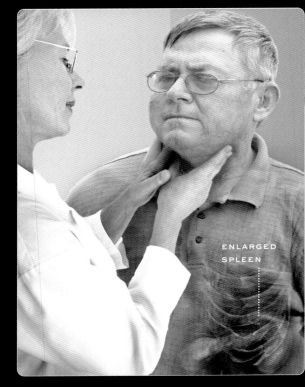

ENLARGED
SPLEEN

GETTING THE WHOLE PICTURE: DIAGNOSING CHRONIC ANEMIA IN CKD

If you are already living with CKD, your doctor will test your blood regularly to check for any possible complications caused by your kidneys' impaired functioning. After a specialist (phlebotomist) draws your blood, the samples are sent to a lab for testing. The tests will involve a complete blood count (CBC), which includes different tests that will help to diagnose anemia. Two major tests in the CBC that show if anemia is present are hematocrit (HCT) or packed cell volume (PCV), and hemoglobin (Hgb).

Hematocrit measures how much of the blood, by volume, is taken up by RBCs. A normal range for hematocrit is 41 to 50 percent in men and 36 to 44 percent in women.

The hemoglobin test measures the amount of hemoglobin molecules in the blood and is a good indicator of the body's ability to carry oxygen throughout the body. A normal range for hemoglobin is 13 to 17 gm/dL in men and 12 to 15 gm/dL in women.

In many cases, a reading below the normal range for both hematocrit and hemoglobin will lead to a diagnosis of CKD-related anemia. If an iron deficiency is found, treatment with iron replacement therapy will begin immediately. If the anemia is serious, treatment with synthetic EPO may also be recommended.

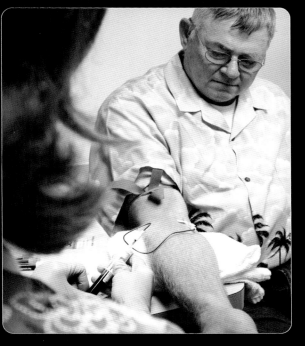

WHAT TO EXPECT WHEN YOU'RE BEING TESTED FOR ANEMIA

When your doctor suspects you might have anemia, you can expect him or her to examine you, checking for swollen lymph nodes, an enlarged spleen, pale skin and changes in nail color. Your blood will also be drawn and sent to a laboratory for various tests.

THE COMPLETE BLOOD TEST, CBC

In a CBC test all the various types of cells that compose the blood are measured and examined. There are six tests in a CBC:

- red blood cell (RBC) count
- hematocrit (density/packing of RBCs)
- hemoglobin
- white blood cell (WBC) count
- differential blood count or the "diff"
- platelet count

TWO CRITICAL BLOOD TESTS

The hematocrit and the hemoglobin are the central tests to diagnosing anemia in that they indicate both the amount of RBCs and hemoglobin in the blood. Interestingly it takes only about one drop of your blood examined under a microscope to calculate the hematocrit.

THE READINGS FOR YOUR HEMOGLOBIN TEST WILL BE ROUGHLY 1/3 OF YOUR HEMATOCRIT NUMBER.

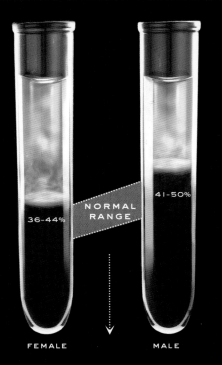

NORMAL RANGE

36-44%

41-50%

FEMALE

MALE

GETTING AN ACCURATE CKD DIAGNOSIS

Chronic kidney disease develops over time. If you have diabetes or hypertension, certain anemias or have a hereditary predisposition to kidney disease, your primary care physician will carefully monitor you for abnormal kidney function. Otherwise, testing for CKD begins when some sign or symptom of kidney abnormality is detected. Unfortunately, you may not experience symptoms until you are already in advanced stages of CKD.

CKD may make you feel very tired and you may have significantly less energy than normal. Other symptoms of CKD include poor appetite, difficulty sleeping, cramping at night, dry itchy skin, swollen feet or ankles, puffiness around your eyes (especially in the morning), trouble concentrating, and the need to urinate more often, especially at night.

Your doctor will screen you for CKD by measuring your blood pressure and testing for substances that should not normally be in the urine and the blood.

URINE ALBUMIN: This test checks for a specific protein, albumin, in the urine. Proteins, necessary for the building and repair of tissues in your body, leak into the urine when the kidney is damaged. "Proteinuria" is the clinical term for having too much protein in your urine.

SERUM CREATININE: This blood test measures how well the kidneys are removing creatinine from your body by calculating how much creatinine is in your blood. The normal creatinine range is 0.6 to 1.2 mg/dL.

CREATININE CLEARANCE (CRCL): This test analyzes renal function by measuring levels of creatinine in your blood compared to levels in your urine. This tells you how fast your kidneys remove creatinine from your body. Creatinine clearance can give an estimation of glomerular filtration rate (GFR), the major indicator of kidney function.

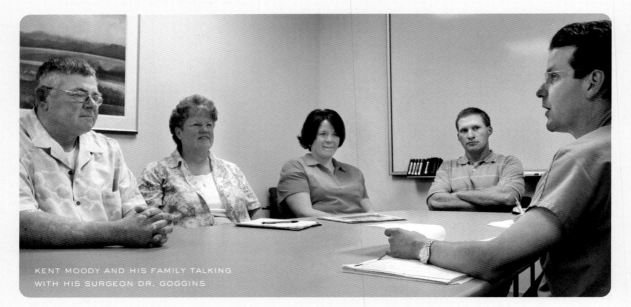

KENT MOODY AND HIS FAMILY TALKING WITH HIS SURGEON DR. GOGGINS

GLOMERULAR FILTRATION RATE (GFR): The GFR gives your doctor the most accurate assessment of overall kidney function. The GFR is figured from an equation that includes factors such as serum creatinine, age, race and gender.

BLOOD UREA NITROGEN (BUN): The BUN measures levels of urea nitrogen in the blood. If it is high, it is another indication of possible kidney disease.

Images can tell their own story and sometimes doctors will order scans in order to visually examine the appearance of the kidneys. The health of your kidneys may also be evaluated by testing the actual tissue.

ULTRASOUND OR CT SCAN: Such screenings may be used to determine abnormalities in kidney size and/or placement, to estimate residual urine, or to pinpoint abnormalities like kidney stones.

KIDNEY BIOPSY: Your doctor will remove small pieces of kidney tissue with a long, thin needle, and then examine them under a microscope. Because of the kidney's intricate network of blood vessels, physicians who biopsy

the kidney rely on an ultrasound machine or a CT scanner to guide the biopsy needle away from large arteries or veins, aiming the needle into the outermost cortex of the kidney. This lessens the chance of complications, such as bleeding, while sampling the part of the kidney containing the most clinically relevant information.

In most cases a nephrologist is called in when moderate kidney damage is apparent, but if you have pre-existing, poorly managed diabetes or hypertension you may be referred to a specialist earlier.

POSSIBLE SYMPTOMS OF CHRONIC KIDNEY DISEASE
• changes in urination patterns
• swelling (edema) of the legs, feet, hands, and/or face
• exceptional fatigue
• itching and possible skin rash
• a metallic taste in the mouth and resulting bad breath
• shortness of breath
• possible nausea and resultant vomiting
• dizziness and trouble concentrating
• leg pain and the sensation of being cold (shivers)

THE STAGES OF CHRONIC KIDNEY DISEASE
There are five stages in the progress of CKD; the first four involve evaluations that still include kidney function. The fifth is actual kidney failure.

STAGE	DESCRIPTION	GLOMERULAR FILTERATION RATE (GFR) (ML/MIN)
1	Kidney damage with normal GFR	> 90
2	Mild decrease in GFR	60–89
3	Moderate decrease in GFR	30–59
4	Severe decrease in GFR	15–29
5	Kidney failure	< 15—or dialysis

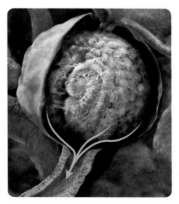

ARROW REPRESENTS DIRECTION OF FILTRATION

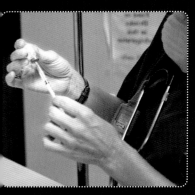

NURSE PREPARING TO ADMINIS-
TER ESA THERAPY (ARTIFICIAL
EPO) TO A PATIENT.

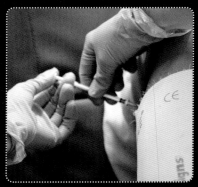

THE INJECTION IS USUALLY GIVEN
UNDER THE SKIN, OR SUBCUTA-
NEOUSLY.

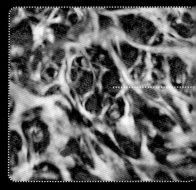

ARTIFICIAL EPO TRAVELS TO THE
BONE MARROW.

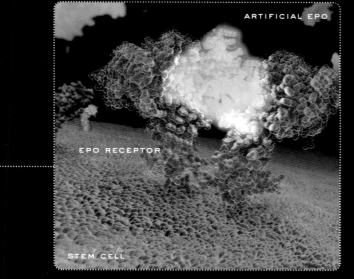

ARTIFICIAL EPO

EPO RECEPTOR

STEM CELL

ARTIFICIAL EPO BINDING TO A
STEM CELL IN THE BONE MARROW

As Kent's CKD progresses, his hemoglobin count, at a low of 10, indicates that he is anemic, characterized by a deficiency of red blood cells. His doctors have decided to administer erythropoietin-stimulating-agent (ESA) therapy because Kent's kidneys cannot supply the EPO needed to stimulate red blood cell production in his bones. The shot gives Kent the EPO he needs, and his hemoglobin count gradually climbs from 10 to 12. Even though he still suffers from CKD, ESA therapy gives Kent so much energy that he refers to the therapy as his "Superman shot."

Until about 45 years ago kidney failure was an outright killer. But the disease lost some of its fatal power when medical scientists found a way to remove toxins from the kidneys with dialysis, a way of filtering the blood without relying on the kidneys. The natural, artful process of waste removal and nutrient replacement in the blood takes place smoothly in the human kidney's nephron. Now, thanks to technology, the same process can be executed by a dialysis machine. Dialysis allows people with temporary kidney failure caused by infection or injury to survive until their kidneys heal. Since its development it has given more than 100,000 people with irreversible kidney damage the ability to live relatively normal lives for years. Dialysis also allows people with CKD to survive while they await transplantation surgery. Today more than 1.5 million patients worldwide rely on dialysis.

A MIRACLE OF MEDICINE: KIDNEY DIALYSIS

HEMODIALYSIS

In hemodialysis, a dialysis machine filters blood from the body as it flows directly from an access point. Creating this portal involves either joining an artery and a vein in the arm to build a fistula, or constructing a shunt. The process itself requires taking "dirty" blood via a tube attached to the fistula or shunt and circulating it through the dialysis machine. Here, artificial membranes, which function much like the nephrons in the kidney, filter and cleanse the blood and return it through the port to the body. There are special fluids in the artificial membrane system of the machine that balance the body's overall chemical and water levels.

PERITONEAL DIALYSIS

Peritoneal dialysis is performed at home and uses the lining of your abdomen, the peritoneum, which is rich in arteries and veins, as a filter. The patient, a family member or a nurse places a specified amount of dialysis fluid into the abdominal cavity through a permanently established access port in the abdomen. The fluid is then left in the system long enough for all the wastes in the blood to be transferred to the dialysis fluid, which is then drained out of the abdomen. The process takes 30-40 minutes, but in most cases must be repeated four times a day.

A NEW KIDNEY

When your kidney can no longer filter blood properly, you will need to consider either dialysis or a kidney transplant. For most people, dialysis is not a satisfactory or long-term solution, since it requires constant and lengthy sessions of being hooked up to the dialysis machine. Before considering a transplant, however, you and your doctor should discuss the preparations needed to find the best match.

WHAT TO EXPECT BEFORE YOUR TRANPLANT

Pre-transplant Evaluation: In order to receive a new kidney, you should be healthy enough to endure the transplant operation, which can take several hours. Your doctor will evaluate your health by performing a physical exam; he will make sure that you are not battling an infection, and will order a chest X-ray to ensure that your lungs and lower GI tract are clear and healthy. He will also ask for an electrocardiogram (EKG or ECG) to see if your heart can handle the oper-

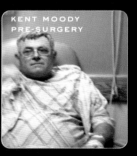

KENT MOODY
PRE-SURGERY

ation. Finally, he will also study an ultrasound of your abdomen and kidneys to assess the condition of your blood vessels, particularly the iliac vessels, which will connect your circulatory system to the new kidney.

THE KIDNEY TRANSPLANT PROCEDURE

As the Living Donor: Your procedure will take place in a separate, but nearby room from the recipient. You will be placed under general anesthesia. Once your kidney is removed, it will be placed on ice and immediately delivered to the recipient's room.

As the Recipient: Once you are placed under general anesthesia, your surgeon will make an incision on the right or left side of the abdomen just above the groin. The donor kidney will be washed with a solution and then placed into your abdomen, where doctors connect it to your iliac artery and vein. Once these sutures are made, the surgeon will then complete the transplant by hooking up the kidney's ureter to your bladder.

LAPAROSCOPY, A MINIMALLY INVASIVE SURGERY

In the last decade, laparoscopic surgery, which requires only small incisions, has replaced conventional operations for kidney removal that used to require a larger opening and therefore longer recovery time. The procedure for living donors involves inserting a special needle into the abdominal cavity to fill it up with gas and create space. A metal tube with a camera, called a laparoscope, is inserted through a two-inch incision in the skin. Surgical instruments can be inserted through the laparoscope, and the surgeon can watch his progress in removing the kidney on a video monitor above the patient. With laparoscopic surgery, donors feel less pain after the transplant, and are able to return to their daily routine sooner.

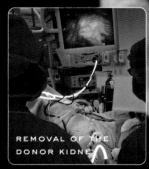

REMOVAL OF THE
DONOR KIDNEY

DISEASED KIDNEYS

TRANSPLANTED
KIDNEY

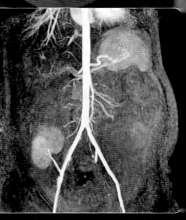

MRI OF TRANSPLANTED
KIDNEY IN PELVIS

URETER

DONOR RENAL
ARTERY

DONOR RENAL
VEIN

DONOR URETER

LIAC ARTERY

LIAC VEIN

The surgery begins with both Adam, the
donor, and Kent, the recipient, in different rooms. In one room, the surgery
team removes Adam's kidney. Adam's
kidney is immediately placed in a bowl
of ice and transported to Kent's surgery
room. As the surgeons place Adam's
kidney into Kent's pelvis and connect it
to his arteries and veins, they watch the
"super kidney" turn crimson red as
Kent's blood rushes in.

82

THE CLOSEST
BOND

Every scar tells a story, and the neat suture running along Kent Moody's abdomen is no exception. After learning that her father needed a new kidney, and that a male's kidney would be ideal, Moody's daughter Christie asked her husband Adam to get tested, to see if he might be a good match. "It wasn't a perfect match but it was the next thing to it," says Moody. "We didn't know they went to get tested, but they came one evening and said that Adam would like to donate

his kidney. I'm very grateful. It's just so great that it overwhelms you in every which way."

Adam turned out to be an ideal donor—young, healthy and willing to give his father-in-law a remarkable gift. With that gift, Moody now has three kidneys; "I have two that aren't too good, and I have one that is a super kidney," he says. The new organ is making a huge difference in Moody's life. His blood sugars and blood pressure have dropped significantly, and most remarkably, just three weeks following the surgery, he shed about 30 pounds of water weight, all excess fluid that he was carrying that should have been filtered out by his kidneys. "I could tell in the hospital that my energy level was going up," he says. "It just turned me around so much that there's no comparison [between] what I thought [would happen] and what has happened and how quickly it happened."

Moody's pill count has dropped too, although he has had to add medication to help him to accept Adam's kidney and not reject the organ. Little by little, Moody's body is coming back into balance, back to a healthier state in which his blood counts are closer to normal, and his blood pressure and blood sugar levels are under control. He watches what he eats, avoiding fried foods and salt, but he is easing back into his active lifestyle. "I'm checking the fields and the grain elevators, but I take it easy. It's a chance of a lifetime and I don't want to mess it up."

WHAT YOU NEED TO KNOW ABOUT BECOMING A KIDNEY DONOR

In the U.S. nearly 74,000 people are waiting for a kidney transplant, but only about 13,000 are donated each year. In Europe nearly 40,000 patients are on organ transplant waiting lists. That's why the celebrities on the following pages, all of whom suffered from kidney disease and were fortunate enough to find a donor, have become passionate about urging people to become organ donors. If you are considering becoming a donor, here are some questions that you should consider:

Q: CAN I BE A LIVING DONOR?
A: You may be eligible to become a donor if you are between 18-60 years of age, are healthy, and do not have cancer or any infections.

Q: WHAT ARE THE ADVANTAGES OF LIVING DONOR ORGANS VS. DECEASED, OR CADAVERIC, DONOR ORGANS?
A: Living donor transplants have higher success rates than cadaveric donor transplants because the living donor kidney can usually be a closer genetic match to the person with kidney disease. The living organ also starts to work immediately, whereas the non-living kidney may take some time before it starts to function. Patients receiving living donor kidneys often require less anti-rejection medication, and, perhaps most importantly, they can plan when and where they will have the transplant.

Q: DO I HAVE TO BE A RELATIVE OF THE PERSON WAITING FOR A KIDNEY TRANSPLANT?

A: No, even unrelated friends or relatives can become donors. But in most cases, living donors are parents, siblings, sons or daughters since they are most likely to have the closest kidney match.

Q: WHAT ARE THE RISKS IF I WERE TO DONATE?
A: Any invasive surgery carries risks, and the donation procedure carries no more risk than any other major operation. The process requires a seven-to-ten-day stay in the hospital after surgery, and most donors are able to return to work in two to six weeks. There may be some pain following the surgery, which can be controlled with medication and proper follow-up treatment to ensure that your body heals normally.

One thing doctors are increasingly asking donors to consider is the longer term consequences of living with one kidney. For the most part, a single healthy kidney can keep your body healthy on its own, but as you age, maintaining that balance—and keeping your blood pressure under control—becomes harder. So as a kidney donor, you should be extra vigilant about eating a healthy diet and staying active.

Q: HOW DO I BECOME A KIDNEY DONOR?
A: In the U.S. the process varies by state, but the easiest way to become a donor is to indicate your desire to do so when you renew your driver's license. In many European countries it is possible to register to donate online at a donor registration website or by carrying an organ donor card.

"I think the most important thing I want people to know is how important it is to be a donor....How many people are sitting right now on a donating list and how many people will never get that chance to be donated to?"
-Carson Kainer

CARSON'S NEW CHANCE

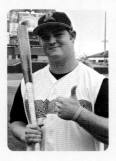

As a college baseball player, Carson Kainer was accustomed to aching muscles, swollen feet, and always feeling exhausted. But Kainer's discomfort came from more than just training to become a professional ball player. Born with chronic renal failure, he had relied on the work of one kidney for most of his life. But in 2006, after 21 years, that organ too was failing, no longer able to filter out toxins from his blood. Just as he had finally realized his dream of joining a professional baseball team, the Cincinnati Reds, Kainer learned he would need a transplant or never play ball again.

Fortunately Kainer's father, who had passed his love of baseball on to his son, was willing to give him one more gift—a healthy kidney. Ten months after the transplant, Kainer returned to the baseball diamond—healthy, eager and now able to endure the rigorous training required of a professional athlete. He is also passionate about educating people about the importance of organ donation. "I want people to know how important it is to be a donor," he says. "I've been given this dona-tion, but I want to show people: look what I've done with my chance, my second chance at life."

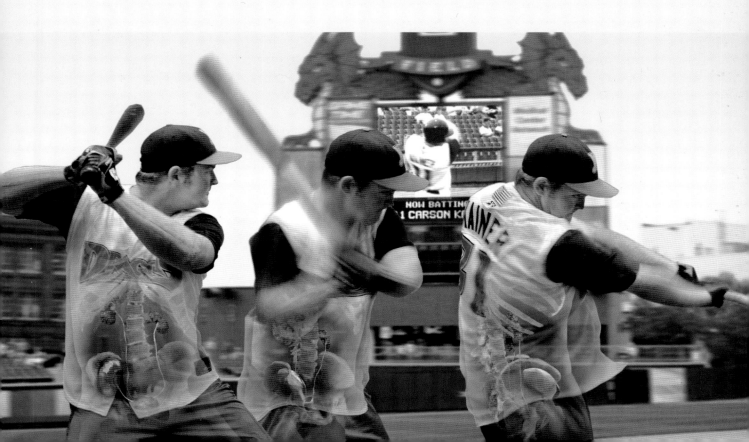

CELEBRITY KIDNEY TRANSPLANT STORIES

COMPATIBILITY TESTING

If a patient passes the health tests, the next step is to find a good match between the donor kidney and the person waiting for a transplant. A match is determined by a number of factors that will be evaluated in a series of tests called histocompatibility (HC) testing. HC testing makes sure the donor and recipient have compatible blood types, that their immune systems are not over active and that they both have similar tissue, or HLA, typing. In tissue typing, genetic markers, or antigens, are identified on the white blood cells of the donor and the kidney patient. Each person inherits these markers from his or her parents, and some antigens are more common than others. The tests will rate the compatibility of the donor or recipient's antigens. For example, an exact match is rated a "6," but even "4" or "5" ratings are sufficient for a transplant.

SEAN ELLIOTT

(ex-pro basketball player)

For any professional basketball player, winning the national championship represents the culmination of their athletic career. For Sean Elliott, a forward with the San Antonio Spurs, however, that milestone only marked the beginning of a more important journey. Just a month after earning the National Basketball Association title with his teammates in 1999, Elliott underwent a kidney transplant with an organ donated from his older brother Noel. Elliott had struggled with focal segmental glomerular sclerosis, a progressive deterioration of his kidney function, for six years; his hands and feet had become increasingly swollen, he had lost his appetite, and he found it more and more difficult to even get out of bed. But thanks to Noel, Elliott returned to the court just seven months after his surgery, becoming the first professional athlete to return to the game following a kidney transplant. Now a broadcaster for the Spurs, Elliott is committed to raising awareness about organ donation and being a living model for others struggling with kidney disease.

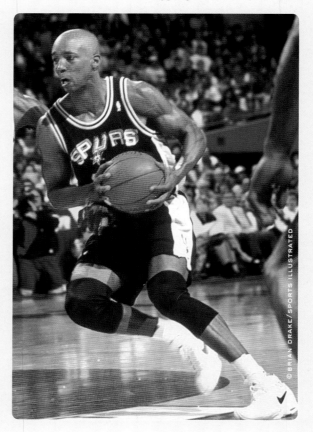

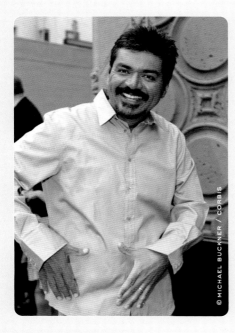

GEORGE LOPEZ
(comedian)

"I'll give you one of mine," Ann Lopez, wife of comedian George Lopez, said as soon as they found out that George was going to need a kidney transplant. "There was no question," Ann told *Primetime* about her decision to donate her kidney to her husband. "When you are put in that position where you could possibly lose someone you love, it's a very easy decision."

When doctors told George that he would need to have transplant surgery, he had 24 episodes of *The George Lopez Show* left to shoot and a demanding tour schedule. "Man, I'm dying,' he recalls telling Ann. "But I love the show, and I'm responsible for 170 people's lives and livelihoods."

George has lived with damaged kidneys his whole life. He was born with a congenital abnormality that caused his ureters, the tubes that transport urine from the kidneys to the bladder, to narrow. As a child, George frequently wet his bed and suffered from the shame this caused his family, who could not, at the time, understand George's medical condition. Later, in his teens, George was diagnosed with hypertension but it wasn't until years later that he began to feel fatigued, even during daily tasks. Still, George refused to see a doctor. "Latinos, we only go to the doctor when we are bleeding," he says with his characteristic humor. "We forget about things internal. Fatigue is just fatigue."

As George finished shooting the remaining episodes of *The George Lopez Show*, Ann underwent various tests to prove that she was in fact a potential match to donate to her husband. She hired a personal trainer to help her get into the best shape possible for the surgery, and shed 15 pounds, meeting with her trainer three days a week.

George barely escaped dialysis, but at the time of the transplant, his kidneys had become so damaged and shrunken that they did not even show up on ultrasound. On April 25, 2005, George and Ann were prepped for surgery in neighboring rooms. Ann's surgery lasted two and a half hours, while George's more complicated procedure took five. The transplant was a success, and though the couple lay recovering in separate rooms, they talked to each other on the phone, relieved to have gotten through the ordeal together.

Three weeks later, George Lopez was playing golf, his favorite pastime. The pain and fatigue were gone. "Even when you know you're going to be well, you don't [anticipate] how well you're going to be," he says. "It's a totally new experience, being healthy. It was like being woken up. I was so toxic. I felt toxic."

Now, healthy and enjoying every minute of his new vitality, George has set his sights on educating others. Both George and Ann have been named spokespeople for the National Kidney Foundation. With one in nine American adults unknowingly suffering from CKD, the foundation hopes that George's popularity, humor and personal experience will help them reach out and educate others with a message he holds dear. He advocates the importance of taking care of one's kidneys and understanding that diseases such as hypertension are very serious and, if not taken care of, can lead to kidney disease. "If laughter is the best medicine," George says to America, "I promise to continue to make you laugh as my wife and I work together with the National Kidney Foundation to save lives."

5

TAKE CARE OF YOUR KIDNEYS; TAKE CARE OF YOUR BLOOD

This chapter is your guide to improving your diet and boosting your level of physical activity. Both are critical factors in improving health and vitality, and this is as true for people who have already developed CKD as it is for individuals who are at risk for developing kidney problems later. CKD patients should ask their doctors to recommend a registered dietician to help them plan the details of their diets, but what follows is information that everyone should be able to put to good use.

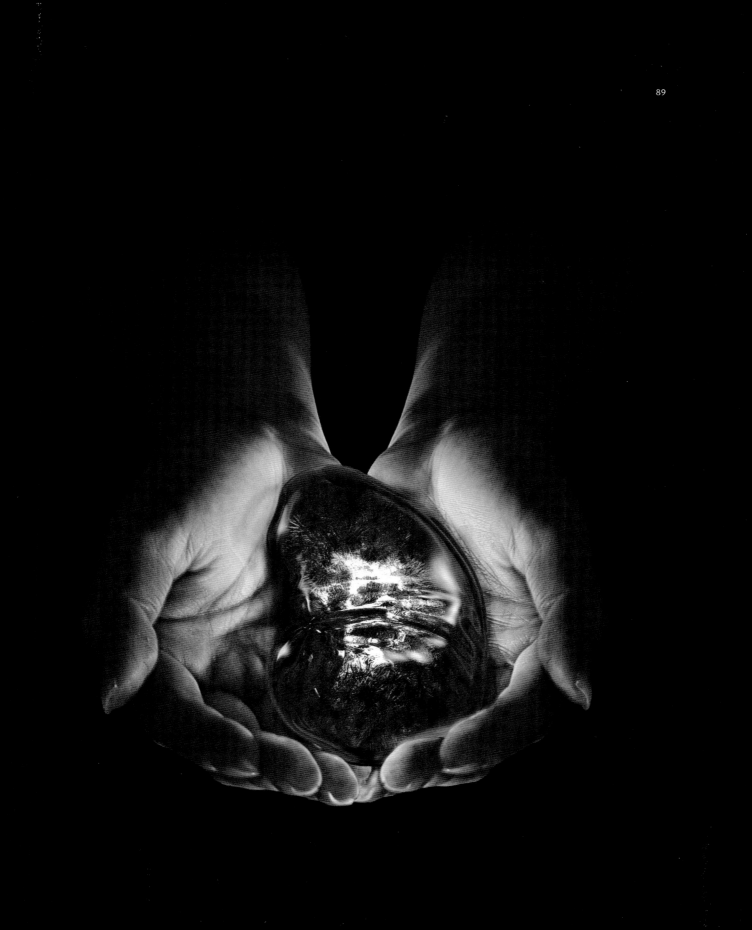

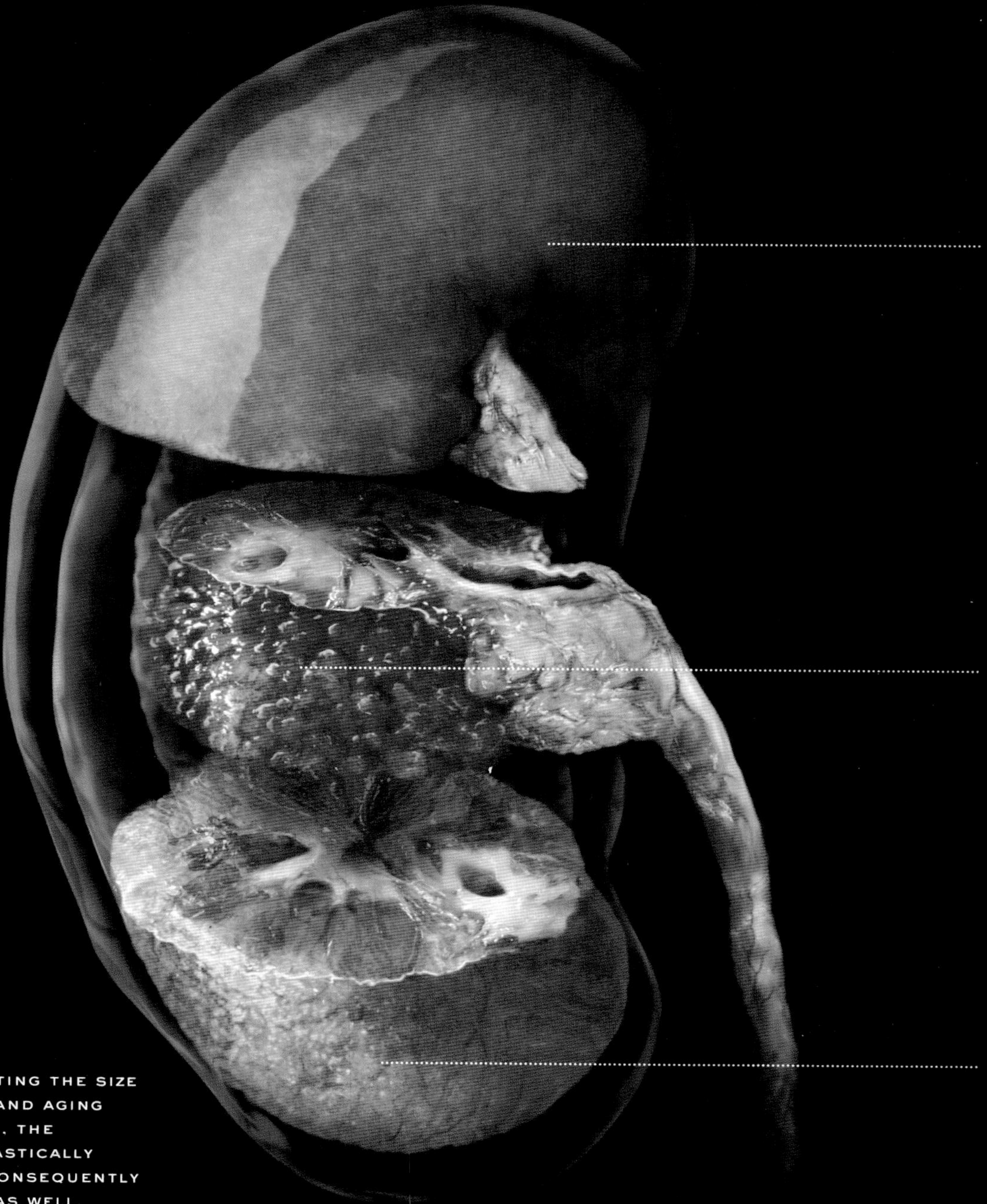

90

HEALTHY KIDNEY

CHRONIC KIDNEY
DISEASE
(HYPERTENSION)

NATURALLY
AGING KIDNEY

GLASS SHELL REPRESENTING THE SIZE
OF THE NORMAL ADULT AND AGING
KIDNEY. IN COMPARISON, THE
DISEASED KIDNEY IS DRASTICALLY
REDUCED IN SIZE AND CONSEQUENTLY
REDUCED IN FUNCTION AS WELL.

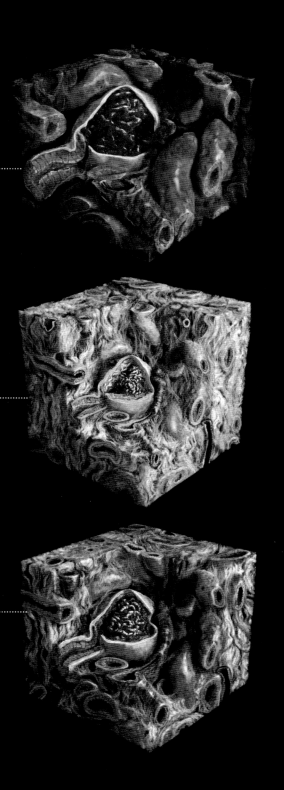

STAYING HEALTHY INSIDE AND OUT

Beauty may be only skin deep, but health certainly isn't. In fact, the opposite is true: the healthier you are on the inside—and this means your heart, your blood, your kidneys and all of your other internal organs—the younger you will look and feel on the outside. But most importantly, the healthier you are, the better you will feel.

As you age, your metabolism slows down. This is why, after about age 40, it is so much harder to lose weight. Most men and women gain about a pound a year, which means that our battle to stay trim just gets more difficult. Additionally, the heart's pumping efficiency decreases, which means that blood flow decreases as well. As you age, your kidneys age with you. The number of nephrons, the kidneys' vital filters, also decreases, as does the overall amount of tissue in the kidneys.

A healthy aging kidney, then, will not function like a 20-year-old kidney, but it can still do its job. The difference between an aging kidney in a healthy body and a kidney damaged by hypertension or diabetes can be as stark as the difference between a picture of health and one of debilitating illness.

THE KIDNEY'S GLOMERULI
(FROM TOP TO BOTTOM)

THE HEALTHY GLOMERULUS FUNCTIONS AT FULL CAPACITY, ENSURING THE BODY'S WASTES ARE FILTERED OUT AND FLUIDS AND ELECTROLYTES ARE BALANCED.

THE DISEASED GLOMERULUS SHOWS DISTINCT SHRINKAGE AS WELL AS A BUILDUP OF CONSTRICTIVE SCAR TISSUE (SCLEROSIS) AND FIBROUS CONNECTIVE TISSUE THAT IMPEDES FUNCTION.

THE AGING GLOMERULUS SHOWS SCLEROSIS, LEADING TO LOSS OF FUNCTION. THE AMOUNT OF ATROPHY VARIES HIGHLY BETWEEN INDIVIDUALS.

NUTRITION FOR THE CKD PATIENT

If you have been diagnosed with CKD, one of the most important things you can do is to carefully watch what you eat. Different foods have different amounts of chemical compounds. Some are high in sugar or fat or vitamin C, for example, while others are high in calcium, sodium or iron. When these different foods are digested, different kinds and amounts of wastes are produced. And this, in turn, can either raise or lower the levels of these wastes in the bloodstream. Because a CKD patient's kidneys cannot effectively remove wastes from the bloodstream, a special diet can help minimize the buildup of those wastes and thereby decrease the workload on the kidneys.

The exact diet CKD patients should follow will depend on the diagnosis and stage of their disease. That is why it is essential to talk to your doctor about getting a dietary plan from a registered dietician who specializes in kidney disease. What may be difficult to understand is why certain foods are labeled good or bad for a kidney patient. Unlike nutritional advice given to the general public to eat more fruits and vegetables, for example, the advice to a CKD patient will be much more specific.

Certain foods may be allowed in early stages of the disease, but could be restricted in later stages. Blood tests will help guide these recommendations. Patients will also need to carefully read labels of prepared foods for the amounts of various ingredients and learn to navigate menus when dining out.

It may at first be confusing and frustrating to be told that a perfectly nutritious fruit, vegetable or other food is actually something you should avoid. But understanding why specific compounds in food can cause further kidney damage will help make these restrictions make sense. Without dietary controls, the disease will progress faster and become more severe. By following dietary restrictions, patients can play a key role in extending and improving the quality of their lives.

SALT

It is essential to life, but because our bodies are built to crave salt, modern diets often include too much. The kidneys balance the amount of salt and fluid in the body in order to maintain proper blood pressure. When healthy people eat too much salt, their bodies adjust and the kidneys excrete more sodium. But when the kidneys are damaged, they are less able to excrete sodium so that even normal salt intake can result in an increase in the fluid retained by the body, which causes blood pressure to rise. Controlling salt is key to controlling hypertension. And because hypertension is the factor that can destroy kidney function most rapidly, restricting salt intake is an important dietary restriction in nearly all CKD patients.

HIGH SODIUM FOODS TO AVOID: table salt, potato chips, bacon, pickles, olives, hot dogs, pastrami, cheese

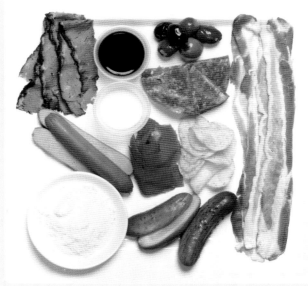

For more information on chronic kidney disease, contact the National Kidney Foundation at www.kidney.org or call toll-free at 800.622.9010.

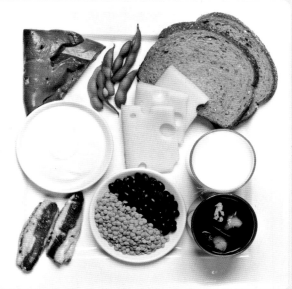

PHOSPHORUS

Phosphorus and calcium work together in close balance to keep bones healthy. But when damaged kidneys cannot remove excess phosphorus from the bloodstream, calcium leaches out of bones to bind with the excess phosphorus. This, in turn, can leave bones weakened. Calcium pulled into the bloodstream from bones can also lead to dangerous deposits in blood vessels, lungs, eyes and the heart. Avoiding foods that are high in phosphorus, such as dairy, can help to prevent this mineral from accumulating in the blood. In some cases, CKD patients take a phosphate binder with their meals to limit how much phosphorus the body absorbs.

HIGH PHOSPHORUS FOODS TO AVOID: beer, dark colas, cheese, milk, pudding, ice cream, beef liver, chicken liver, oysters, sardines, baked beans, lentils, soy beans, kidney beans, bran cereals, nuts, seeds, whole grain products

POTASSIUM

This mineral, found in a large variety of foods, plays an important role in keeping your heartbeat regular and your muscles working. High potassium levels can be very dangerous, but usually only in advanced kidney disease. Symptoms can include weak muscles, irregular heartbeat or a heart attack. Because potassium is found in foods such as whole grains that many diabetics depend on, restriction of this mineral can be modified to meet the particular dietary needs of the CKD patient. It is important to note that many salt substitutes often contain large amounts of potassium and should also be avoided.

HIGH POTASSIUM FOODS TO AVOID: avocado, banana, orange, beets, broccoli, brussel sprouts, carrots (raw), lentils, spinach, tomatoes, nuts/seeds, peanut butter, yogurt

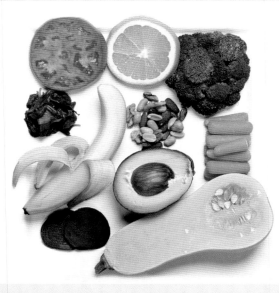

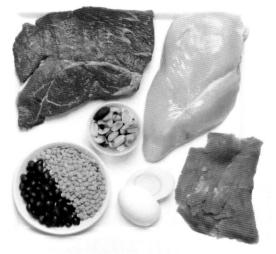

PROTEIN

When your body digests protein, a waste product called urea is produced. If kidney function is diminished, this waste can build up in the blood and cause fatigue and loss of appetite. CKD patients are usually placed on a modest protein restriction (a phosphorus reduction, since phosphorus is found in dairy protein, usually also results in lower protein in the diet). In some patients a low-protein diet can improve symptoms like nausea or vomiting. There isn't as much evidence, however, that even lower protein levels in the diet slow the progression of the disease. And too little protein can result in malnourishment, which can be an even worse problem for a CKD patient.

SUPPLEMENTS

Billions of dollars are spent each year on herbal supplements as people try to find complementary approaches to medical treatment. And there are certainly potent and potentially useful chemical compounds in traditional botanical treatments. But there is little regulation of their purity, safety or effectiveness. And even herbal products that might be safe in healthy people could pose a risk to patients with CKD because of their vulnerable kidney function. The safest course is to talk to your doctor before taking any herbal supplement.

MAY BE TOXIC IN CKD: alfalfa, blue cohosh, capsicum, dandelion, ginseng, licorice, mate, nettle, noni juice, rhubarb, sassafras, vervain

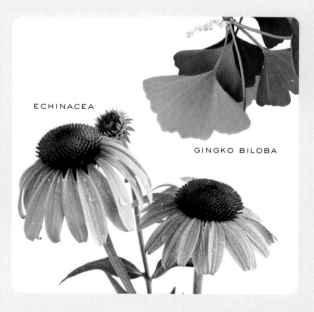

ECHINACEA

GINGKO BILOBA

WHAT IT TAKES: HEALTHY DIET HABITS HELP MANAGE CKD

Poor eating habits are taking a terrible toll across the world. At least 20 million children under the age of 5 years and more than 1.6 billion adults are overweight, with 400 million of them qualifying as obese. The medical consequences are also enormous. Eight out of 10 cases of Type 2 diabetes and cardiovascular disease are related to unhealthy eating and lifestyle habits.

It is easy to say that we eat too much and exercise too little, but it is also easy to understand why. We live in a fast food world where we are constantly tempted by the very foods that are bad for us. Making matters worse, it is biologically natural for us to love foods that are loaded with salt, sugar and fats. Our prehistoric ancestors had no guarantees where or when they would find their next meal. Their bodies developed certain traits that helped them survive. When they found foods rich in calories and nutrients, it was smart for them to eat as much of those as they could. And because food was often scarce, it was also smart for them to keep eating even after they were full.

In much of the world today, however, food is cheap and plentiful. Our bodies, unfortunately, are still hostage to our prehistoric heritage. Even countries that previously had low rates of obesity are adopting more "western" lifestyles, particularly in urban areas, making them more susceptible to risk factors such as diabetes and hypertension. No wonder we struggle with our weight. But because obesity plays such a role in so many of the diseases that are also associated with kidney disease, taking steps to lose weight and improve your diet can help you avoid developing kidney disease.

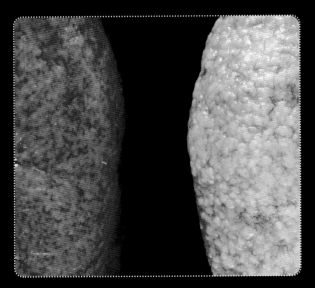

HEALTHY KIDNEY   UNHEALTHY KIDNEY (HYPERTENSIVE)

ENVIRONMENTAL HAZARDS: We live in a time and place where temptation is everywhere. The food industry spends billions of advertising dollars each year to persuade us to eat our fill of the high-fat, high-sugar and salty foods we crave.

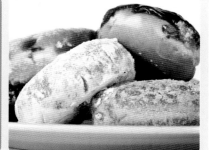

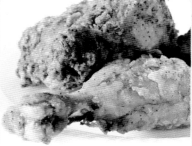

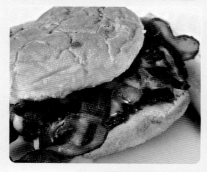

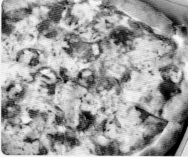

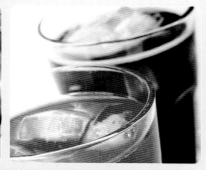

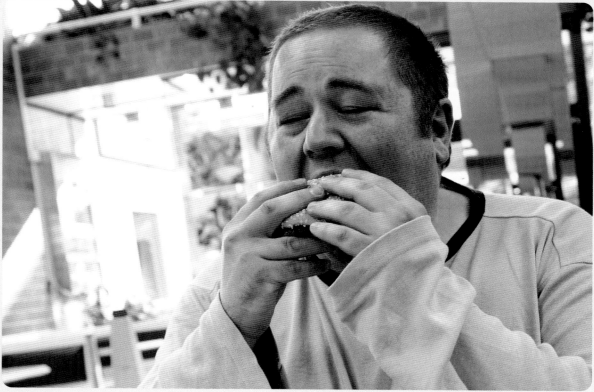

STEP BY STEP: MODIFYING WHAT YOU EAT AND HOW YOU EAT IT

Developing better eating habits happens one meal at a time. The trick is to start by making small changes that you can stick with and build on. First step? Try cutting down on the portions of your favorites; have just half the serving of French fries you'd normally order, for example. Then try substituting healthier choices for those old favorites, like low-fat frozen yogurt instead of ice cream. Meanwhile, find ways to include new, healthy foods and snacks into your daily routine. And remember, even if you are eating at a fast food restaurant, you still have opportunities to make smarter and healthier food choices.

GRAINS

Government dietary advice suggests that at least half of the breads, pasta, rice and other complex carbohydrates we eat come from whole grains. Cut out the highly processed and refined carbohydrates found in snacks, cakes and cookies, which are broken down very quickly by the body. Instead try brown rice, whole wheat bread, and other grains, such as bulgur, wild rice and barley, as side dishes or added to soups. Whole grains are digested more slowly—so you feel full longer—and are also excellent sources of key vitamins, minerals and fiber.

FRUITS AND VEGETABLES

We should be eating five to nine servings of fruits and vegetables each day. And yet, for too many people, a serving of fruit stops at a glass of juice. And recent studies in the U.S. have found that the most popular vegetables are iceberg lettuce, tomatoes (as ketchup or pizza sauce) and French fries. Nutrition experts recommend two cups of fruit and two cups of vegetables each day. In particular, they stress variety, suggesting we eat more dark leafy greens and colorful vegetables, because of the micronutrients they contain.

MEAT, DAIRY, BEANS, AND NUTS

Most nutritionists feel that residents of industrialized countries eat more protein than they need and most of it is from meats and dairy products. Annual meat production is projected to increase from 218 million tons in 1997-1999 to 376 million tons by 2030. Although this may be a positive change in developing countries, the excessive consumption of animal products in the industrialized world is leading to excessive intakes of fat. In these cases, a healthier alternative would be to get dairy protein from low-fat or fat-free milk products and animal protein from leaner cuts of meat. Our diets should also include more fish as well as more plant proteins, such as dried beans, lentils and nuts, since they also are excellent sources of important nutrients and fiber.

OILS AND FATS

Dietary fat helps the body absorb vitamins and nutrients. The key is in choosing the right kind of fats. Too much dietary fat is made up of saturated fats, like those found in butter, meat and certain plant oils like palm and coconut (which are heavily used in processed foods). A healthy diet should include less of those fats and more of the polyunsaturated and monounsaturated fats found in safflower, sunflower, corn, olive, soybean and peanut oils. And trans fats (often labeled "partially hydrogenated oil"), used in margarine, shortenings and in the food industry to fry foods, should be avoided because they raise levels of "bad" cholesterol in your blood.

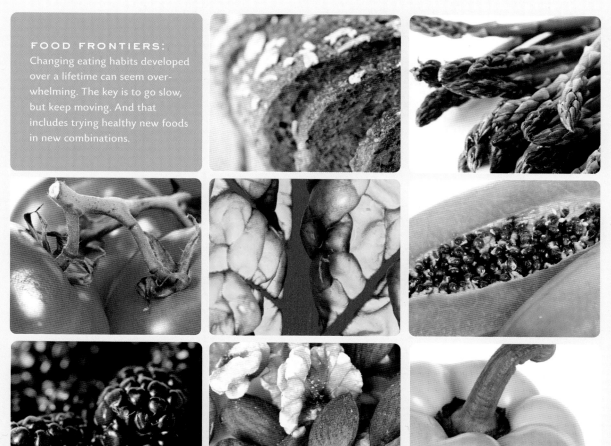

FOOD FRONTIERS:
Changing eating habits developed over a lifetime can seem over-whelming. The key is to go slow, but keep moving. And that includes trying healthy new foods in new combinations.

THE SIMPLE ART OF THE MAIN COURSE SALAD

You can create a whole, nutritious meal without great effort. All you need is to have some cooked chicken on hand, fresh greens, your favorite vegetables—such as peppers, onions, carrots, avocados, and tomatoes. Add your favorite condiments, nuts or seeds. Drizzle on some low-fat dressing, toss and enjoy. Vary the routine by using black beans, canned tuna or other healthy leftovers.

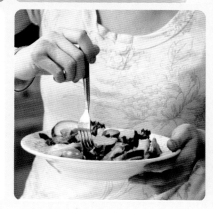

WATER, THE GREATEST DRINK ON EARTH

Your kidneys need to produce enough urine to facilitate waste removal from the body, and for this reason an adequate intake of water is essential; at least eight cups (each an eight-ounce serving) daily.

Too little water is the most common problem, but sometimes hyperhydration (too much water) can also be a concern. In certain cases, drinking too much water (or receiving too much fluid intravenously) can cause sodium levels in the blood to drop dangerously low, a condition called hyponatremia.

HOW MUCH WATER IS GOOD FOR YOU?

You lose water via perspiration, urine, bowel movements, and even your breath. This water must be replaced for your body to function properly. Foods account for about 20 percent of total fluid intake, so foods that have high water content, like fruits and vegetables (melons, strawberries, apples, pears, cucumbers, squash, green vegetables) are especially good for this purpose. As long as you also consume about eight cups of water (two liters) or other beverages per day, you'll keep your fluid level normal. Larger men need about 12 to 13 cups of liquid a day.

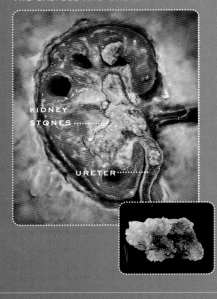

A CROSS-SECTIONED KIDNEY SHOWING KIDNEY STONES WITHIN THE CALYCES AND URETER.

KIDNEY STONES

URETER

WATER IS THE BEST DEFENSE AGAINST KIDNEY STONES, JUST ONE CAUSE OF CKD

If you have had a kidney stone or know you are at risk for kidney stones, protect yourself by drinking more water, which dilutes the levels of wastes. When urine is less concentrated, there is less chance that kidney stones will form. For some people that might mean three to four quarts throughout the day. And in hot weather, they may need to drink even more to make up for fluid loss from sweating. Most of the fluid should be just water. Alcohol and caffeinated beverages are diuretics, which means that they cause the body to eliminate fluid faster than normal.

Not all kidney stones are the same. The most common types are those that are made of calcium or oxalate. In many cases, further stone formation can be prevented in kidney patients if they follow a special diet. Depending on what sort of stone you are at risk for developing, your doctor may have you cut back on salt and sometimes calcium, or foods high in the compound oxalate, such as peanuts, rhubarb, chocolate, sweet potatoes or spinach.

WATER CAUTION

If you have CKD, however, you should consult your doctor about how much water you should be drinking each day. Depending on the stage of the disease, CKD can cause disturbances in fluid balance and in the levels of electrolytes such as potassium, calcium, sodium and magnesium. In most early stages of CKD, patients are on a liberal fluid intake, but in later stages, fluid might be restricted, and if you are on dialysis, water can be the enemy. Though again, it depends on which type of dialysis a patient is undergoing; most patients are on a very strict fluid restriction.

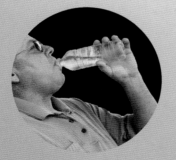

As a renal transplant recipient, Kent Moody must drink at least five liters of water every day to maintain kidney health.

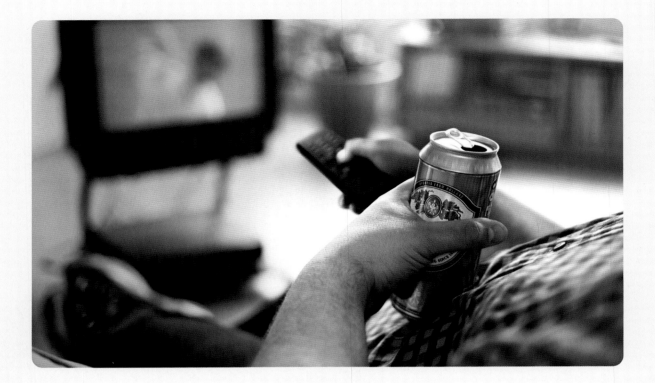

THE BENEFITS OF EXERCISE: MOVE IT AND LOSE IT

Calories may seem old-fashioned, but they still count. If you eat and drink more calories than your body burns, you will gain weight, whether those calories are from heart-healthy dishes or fast food meals. Part of the problem is that portion sizes have steadily become bigger. With 25 percent of Americans and 10-20 percent of the world population overweight or obese, we need to cut back on the sheer amount we eat. It isn't just super-sized fries and soft drinks that are the problem. We need to recognize that bottomless bowls of pasta, baskets of breadsticks and even the endless salad bars are also to blame.

The other part of the equation, however, is that we need to burn off more of those calories through exercise. Health experts suggest that adults engage in 60 minutes of moderate to vigorous exercise most days of the week. And that's just to maintain a healthy weight. To lose weight usually takes 60-90 minutes a day. And yet according to recent studies, more than half of U.S. and European adults do not get enough physical activity to provide even minimal health benefits, let alone weight control. One-quarter of adults get virtually no exercise.

NEED MOTIVATION? CONSIDER THIS:
Nearly one million deaths in the U.S. and one out of every five deaths in the European Union each year are preventable through diet and lifestyle changes. One of the leading preventable causes of death and disease is still cigarette smoking, which kills nearly 10 million people each year. But climbing fast are deaths due to poor diet and physical inactivity, deaths which are increasing in both the U.S. and Europe annually.

THE ESSENTIAL: EXERCISE AND CARDIOVASCULAR HEALTH

Despite all the fitness programs, health clubs, and athletic gear that are available to inspire us, we continue to be an unreformed sedentary culture. Blame it on technology or on our idea that the less we have to move the greater progress we have made, but in the end, blame falls on our own shoulders. The good news is that when we get up and moving, changing old habits, we get all the credit, too.

ANAEROBIC OPTIONS

The definition of anaerobic exercise is that it is performed "without oxygen." That doesn't mean, however, exercising while holding your breath; the absence of oxygen is occurring at the molecular level. Because the muscles being exercised don't have sufficient oxygen, they must use alternate pathways to produce energy. Examples of anaerobic exercise include very short bursts of exertion, like weight training. Anaerobic exercise is an important part of overall fitness and nearly everyone can benefit from this type of strengthening and conditioning. Free weights can be used in anaerobic exercise routines that include biceps curls and squats. The weights don't have to be heavy and can be used for short periods of time, several times a day. When you challenge your muscles this way, you trigger the slow burning of blood sugar, improve muscle function, and boost waste transport from muscles through the blood—all of which are very important for someone managing CKD and diabetes at the same time.

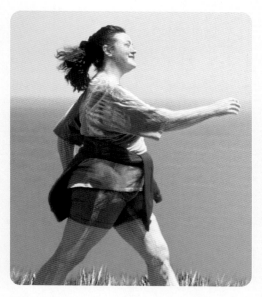

CARDIOVASCULAR TRAINING INCREASES THE STRENGTH OF THE HEART, WHICH IN TURN ALLOWS FOR GREATER BLOOD FLOW THROUGH THE BLOOD VESSELS.

AEROBIC OPTIONS

Aerobic exercise, such as running, swimming and walking, temporarily raises the heart rate, which burns calories. Getting your heart pumping improves healthy oxygen flow through the blood, blood pressure, and resting heart rates. Aerobic exercise strengthens the heart, which is of utmost importance to those living with CKD. It also increases endurance and helps maintain a healthy immune system. Fitting in a cardio workout is as easy as walking. As the philosopher Kierkegaard stated, "Every walk is a good walk." Walking is easy on the joints. You don't have to join a health club or gym. The risk of injury is minimal, and it doesn't require any financial investment beyond a good pair of sneakers or walking shoes.

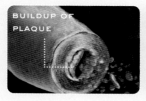

ARTERY OF A SEDENTARY PERSON WITH DECREASED BLOOD FLOW.

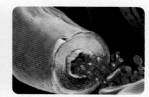

ARTERY OF AN ACTIVE PERSON WITH HEALTHY BLOOD FLOW.

GOING IN THE WRONG DIRECTION: EPO AND BLOOD DOPING

Because EPO is so critical to optimal physical function, some elite athletes have attempted to gain a performance edge by artificially boosting their EPO levels with injections of the hormone. This practice, referred to as blood doping, is seen particularly in endurance sports such as cycling, cross-country skiing and long distance running, for the same reasons that athletes engage in altitude training: the more oxygen the blood can provide, the greater the athlete's stamina and endurance. The International Olympic Committee and many other sports organizations, however, consider artificial EPO boosting unethical and illegal.

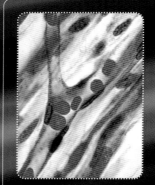

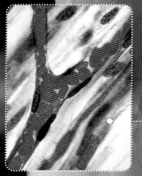

MUSCLE FIBERS

NORMAL RED BLOOD CELL AMOUNT IN CAPILLARY

HIGHER RED BLOOD CELL AMOUNT IN CAPILLARY

BLOOD DOPING CAN CAUSE A DISORDER CALLED POLYCYTHEMIA, A DANGEROUS CONDITION THAT CAN RESULT FROM BONE MARROW CANCER. IT CAN ALSO SOMETIMES OCCUR IN INDIVIDUALS LIVING AT HIGH ALTITUDES, AS THE BODY OVERCOMPENSATES FOR LOWER OXYGEN LEVELS. IN POLYCYTHEMIA THERE IS AN ABNORMAL INCREASE IN TOTAL RED BLOOD CELLS IN THE BODY, WHICH IN TURN INCREASES THE VISCOSITY OF THE BLOOD, CAUSING IT TO FLOW SLUGGISHLY. SYMPTOMS MAY INCLUDE HEADACHES, BLURRED VISION, HIGH BLOOD PRESSURE, DIZZINESS AND NIGHT SWEATS.

A NATURAL WAY TO BOOST RED BLOOD CELL COUNT: HIGH ALTITUDE TRAINING

In order to compete with the best runners in the world, Brandon Leslie trains at high altitude. He travels from his home in Albuquerque, New Mexico (elevation: 5,000 feet above sea level) to the Center for High Altitude Training in Flagstaff, Arizona (elevation: 7,000 feet above sea level), where he trains with other elite runners.

In two to six weeks, the bodies of the runners adjust to their surroundings. The physiological changes that take place are the result of their bodies adapting to an environment in which there is less available oxygen. This means that the amount of oxygen that their RBCs pick up from air in their lungs is reduced.

After just a few days training at the Center, Brandon's kidneys sense the reduced oxygen levels and respond by producing more EPO—which binds to stem cells in the bone marrow and causes more RBCs to be produced. This, in turn, will mean more oxygen can be delivered to his muscles.

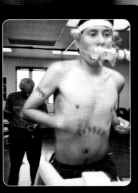

WHILE RUNNING AT MAXIMUM SPEED ON A TREADMILL, BRANDON IS HOOKED UP TO A MACHINE THAT WILL MEASURE HIS MAXIMAL OXYGEN UPTAKE, OR VO2 MAX. ALTITUDE TRAINING SHOULD INCREASE BRANDON'S VO2 MAX.

A POPULAR SEQUENCE
OF YOGA POSES:
SUN SALUTATION

GETTING GOING: GENTLE WAYS TO INTRODUCE EXERCISE TO YOUR LIFE

INTRODUCING GREATER PHYSICAL ACTIVITY INTO YOUR DAILY LIFE

It can be daunting to think about beginning an exercise program if you are out of shape or if you have limited mobility. But making changes in your level of physical activity can be gradual, just like making changes to your diet. Begin with activities you know you can do and then build new activities into your routine. The key is to find your own way to incorporate exercise into your day. For some that might be turning a shopping trip into an exercise opportunity by parking at the far end of the lot and taking the stairs instead of the elevator. For others it might mean taking the dog on an extra walk or renting a beginning exercise video. Exercise doesn't have to feel like gym class. Consider some ancient traditional alternatives that have proven effective for centuries.

YOGA: Yoga can provide overall physical condition-ing, including improved balance and flexibility, as well as the benefits of meditation. Yoga poses and pos-tures and deep breathing techniques can be practiced at home with the aid of a book, tape or DVD. Yoga studios and most gyms offer classes for all levels. Many community centers and even churches are also offering yoga classes, which can be an especially good place for older beginners to be introduced to yoga.

TAI CHI: Tai chi is a traditional Chinese martial art long believed to promote health and longevity. In recent years it has also gained popularity in the U.S. and Europe as a form of exercise and relaxation tech-nique. The core movements in Tai chi are the gentle and slow tracing of circles in the air while shifting the body's weight back and forth from leg to leg. While doing this, you will also be practicing deep breathing techniques. You can find instruction at a Tai chi center or take a class at almost any health club, and like yoga, it is often available at community centers for older adults.

FAMILY AND FRIENDS: GOOD MEDICINE FOR MOTIVATION

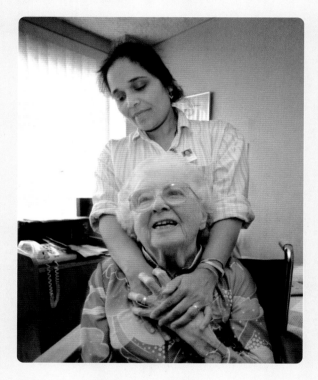

Social support can make a world of difference when you are battling an illness. Your friends and family play a key role. They can help you with the logistics of making medical appointments as well as share in your efforts to begin an exercise program and develop healthier eating habits. They can listen to your concerns, encourage you and help you understand the information you need to effectively manage your illness. They can keep you from feeling overwhelmed.

But support doesn't end with the family. There are many people who are struggling with kidney disease or are at risk for obesity-related disorders who can't rely on family. Thankfully there are a growing number of support networks for these individuals as well. No one will know better what you are going through than other patients. Your hospital or clinic will almost surely have patient groups you can join. Sharing your struggles and successes with other patients can be a source of solace and strength.

Perhaps the most important thing to remember is that even when you feel frustrated or helpless in the face of illness, there are many things you can do to improve the quality of your life. Find ways to cultivate resources and support from your own community.

TO YOUR HEALTH: A NEW BEGINNING

Being healthy is our greatest asset. Good health depends on healthy kidneys. Healthy kidneys depend on healthy blood. The health of both depends on our understanding of how they are intimately related and how they must work together to keep us well.

You have looked into the intricate workings of an extraordinary human engine of health and vitality.

Appreciating the importance of prevention as well as understanding what is involved in treatment and management are the critical first steps. The challenge is to now develop the resources that will enable you to become an active partner in your own health care. You can do it. Take a deep breath. Make it happen.

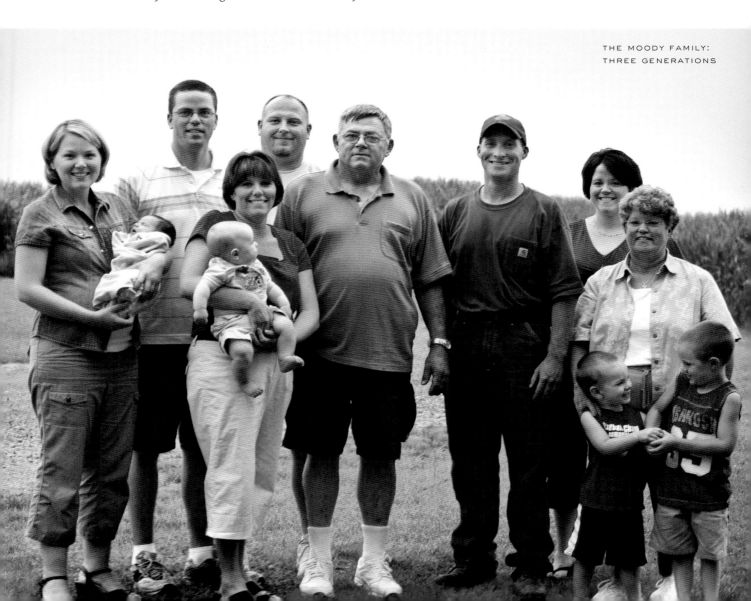

THE MOODY FAMILY:
THREE GENERATIONS

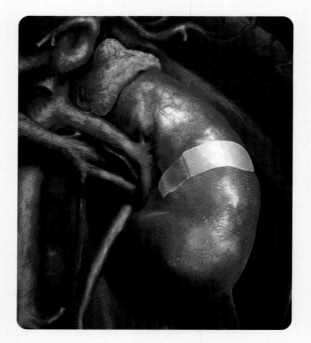

A

Adrenal gland (Suprarenal gland) A small gland (one to two inches long) located on top of each kidney. The adrenal gland secretes hormones that affect the body's metabolism and help a person cope with emotional and physical stress. 24

Afferent arteriole Blood vessel that branches from the interlobular arteries in the kidney and supplies blood to the nephrons. 32, 33, 34

Alveolus (pl. alveoli) Small saclike structure. In the lungs, the alveolus is one of millions of tiny balloon-like structures located at the ends of the bronchioles where oxygen is exchanged for carbon dioxide. Air enters through the nose or mouth, down the trachea, through the bronchi, further into the bronchioles, and finally into the alveoli. 18

Analgesic nephropathy Kidney damage caused by long-term and/or overuse of pain relievers (analgesics). 9

Anemia A condition characterized by a deficiency of RBCs and/or hemoglobin within the RBCs, or reduced volume of blood. Anemic RBCs cannot function adequately to supply oxygen to the body's tissues. viii, xiv, 2, 5, 8-11, 43, 54-63, 66, 72-74, 77

Angiogram A diagnostic imaging test used to visualize blood vessels. Contrast dye is injected through a catheter into the bloodstream, making blood flow visible with an X-ray. 2-3

Aorta The largest artery that arises from the heart. It divides into the arterial system and transports oxygenated blood to the rest of the body. 24

Artery A muscular blood vessel that transports blood away from the heart to the smaller blood vessels throughout the rest of the body. 25, 35, 48, 78, 80, 81, 103

Arteriole Small blood vessels that branch from arteries to capillaries. 32, 33, 34, 47, 48

B

Bilirubin The breakdown product of hemoglobin. It is a pigment that gives bile its distinctive yellow-brown tint and also makes stool brown. 21

Bladder Part of the urinary system, the bladder is a muscular sac into which urine flows from the kidneys through the ureter. As the bladder fills with fluid, nerve fibers in the walls detect stretching and signal the need to void. 24, 25, 32, 70, 80, 87

Blood The fluid connective tissue pumped from the heart through all the arteries, capillaries and veins. It consists of a clear yellow liquid called plasma, red and white blood cells, and platelets. The major function of the blood is to transport oxygen and nutrients to the cells of the body and to remove carbon dioxide and other wastes from the cells. Blood is also important in fighting infection and promoting clotting at wound sites. viii, x-xii, xiv, 1-13, 15-18, 20, 22-26, 32, 35-37, 39, 46, 48, 50-52, 56, 58, 60, 62, 63, 66-70, 72-75, 77-83, 85, 86, 88, 91, 94, 95, 98, 100, 103, 104, 105, 109

Blood doping The illegal technique of increasing oxygen capacity with blood transfusions or synthetic EPO to enhance athletic performance. 104

Blood sugar (see Glucose)

Bone marrow The soft tissue within the cavities of bones that house the body's supply of stem cells. All RBCs, many white blood cells and platelets are produced here. viii, 1, 2, 4, 6, 20-22, 26, 35-39, 54, 61-63, 76, 77, 104, 105

C

Capillary The smallest type of blood vessel in the body, connecting the arterioles and venules. Different types of capillaries vary by location in the body; continuous are found in the muscle, lung and central nervous system; sinusoid are found in the liver, spleen and bone marrow; fenestrated are located in the endocrine glands, the intestine, gallbladder and the kidneys. 1, 2, 4, 18, 19, 23, 32-35, 47, 48, 50, 52, 53, 63, 70, 104

Cardiovascular (Circulatory) system Main components include the heart and all the blood vessels. The system is responsible for circulating blood throughout the body. 56, 80, 103

Chemotherapy Therapies consisting of chemical agents that treat cancer by targeting and destroying cancer cells. Rather than destroying the cells directly, the cytotoxic agents impair the cells' ability to replicate. 11, 60, 61

Chronic kidney disease (CKD) (see Kidney failure)

Chronic kidney failure (CKF) (see Kidney failure)

Cystic kidney disease An inherited disease which causes large cysts to form and expand in the kidneys, resulting in a loss of functional renal tubules. 44

D

Diabetes viii, xiv, 8, 43, 44, 50-52, 56, 65, 66, 68-70, 74, 75, 77, 91, 96, 103

Type I (insulin-dependent or juvenile-onset diabetes) An autoimmune disease that occurs when the pancreas produces little to no insulin, a hormone necessary for the absorption of glucose into the cells. It is usually genetic and is characterized by high levels of blood glucose. Patients typically regulate their blood glucose through insulin injections. 69

Type II (insulin-independent or adult-onset diabetes) A disease that occurs when the body does not produce enough insulin or does not use insulin properly (insulin resistance). It is often associated with obesity. Patients typically treat this disorder with exercise and dietary modifications. 50, 69, 96

E

Edema Swelling that usually occurs in the legs and ankles due to excessive fluid accumulation. It may also occur in other parts of the body as well. 27, 56, 75

Efferent arteriole Blood vessel that continues away from the glomerulus carrying filtered blood. 33, 34

Enlarged (hypertrophied) heart When the heart muscle pumps harder and harder to compensate for the deficiency of RBCs (and thus oxygen) in the body. The site of enlargement is usually the left ventricle because it must send blood throughout the whole body. 57

Erythrocyte (red blood cell, RBC) The major cellular element of the circulating blood, reddish in color and biconcave (indented on both sides) in shape, approximately seven micrometers in diameter, and responsible for oxygen delivery to the body's cells. viii, x-xii, xiv, 1-11, 15-22, 24, 26, 35-41, 54, 57, 61-63, 67, 72, 73, 76, 77, 104, 105

Erythropoietin (EPO) A glycoprotein hormone produced mainly in the kidneys and responsible for triggering RBC production by bone marrow stem cells. It is released into the bloodstream when anoxia (lack of oxygen) occurs. viii, 1-3, 6, 7, 9, 15, 22, 26, 35-37, 39, 54, 57, 58, 61, 67, 72, 76, 77, 104, 105

Erythropoietin receptor The specific cellular protein in the stem/progenitor cell's wall that EPO binds to, intiating hematopoiesis. 37, 77

F

Fenestrated capillary Capillary with fenestrations, or pores, in the endothelial cells of the walls, allowing fluids and substances to pass through. 34, 35, 53

G

Globin The protein component of hemoglobin. 17, 21, 39, 62

Glomerular capsule (Bowman's capsule) The saclike beginning of the nephron enclosing a glomerulus. It collects filtrate from the blood and connects to the proximal tubule. 33-35, 48

Glomerular filtration rate (GFR) The volume of fluid, over time, filtered from the renal glomerular capillaries into the Bowman's capsule. A clinical measurement to determine renal function. x, 15, 74, 75

Glomerular sclerosis An irreversible kidney disease in which most or all function is lost as fibrous scar tissue replaces the glomeruli. 84, 91

Glomerulonephritis A group of diseases that cause inflammation of the kidneys' glomeruli, which may be caused by a systemic disease such as a streptococcal infection. 44

Glomerulus (pl. glomeruli) Vascular component of the nephron housed within the Bowman's capsule, consisting of a tuft that divides into several lobes of fenestrated capillaries. 25, 32-35, 44, 48, 49, 52, 75, 91

Glucometer A portable device used by diabetics to test blood sugar levels on a daily basis. A test strip provides the sugar level reading from one drop of blood. 68

Glucose (blood sugar) A simple carbohydrate, the main energy source in the body, and found in the blood. 44, 50, 52, 67-69, 82, 83, 103

H

Heart attack (myocardial infarction) The death or damage of heart muscle due to oxygen deprivation, commonly caused by the partial or complete blockage of the main arteries of the heart. It is typically preceded by chest pain that radiates to the left arm. 47, 56, 94

Hematocrit The measure of RBCs in the blood. It is expressed as a percentage of the total blood volume. xi, 5, 72, 73

Hematopoiesis Development of blood cells. 1, *40-41*

Heme The red-pigmented, iron-containing, oxygen-binding component of hemoglobin. 17, 21, 39

Hemodialysis The procedure by which wastes and other impurities are removed from the blood by circulating the blood through filters outside of the body in a machine. Patients typically undergo hemodialysis outside of the home three times a week, with each session lasting three to four hours. 78

Hemoglobin A complex protein-iron compound in the RBC responsible for carrying oxygen to the cells. xi, 1, 5, 16, 17, 39, 54, 61-63, 72, 73, 77

Henle's loop (loop of Henle) The U-shaped portion of the nephron, connecting the proximal and distal tubules. 32, 33

Hypertension High blood pressure, or increased prolonged pressure against blood vessel walls. Can cause hardening of the blood vessels and lead to heart disease. viii, xiv, 8, 43, 44, 46, 47-49, 56, 65, 67, 70, 74, 75, 87, 90, 91, 93, 96

I

Insulin The hormone produced by the pancreas that enables the body's cells to take in glucose for energy, helping to maintain unharmful levels in the bloodstream. 44, 50, 51, 67, 69, 77

Iron The element (and metal) that oxygen binds to in the hemoglobin of RBCs. 1, 17, 21, 62, 67, 72, 77, 92

J

Juxtaglomerular apparatus A collection of cells, which include the macula densa and juxtaglomerular cells, near the vascular pole of the glomerular capsule that help the nephron regulate renal blood pressure. 32, 33

Juxtaglomerular cells (JG cells or granular cells) Cells lining the afferent arteriole that communicate with the macula densa and create, store and secrete renin to regulate blood pressure. 32, 33

K

Kidney One of a pair of bean-shaped organs located in the posterior abdomen, one on each side of the spine. Each kidney is composed of more than one million nephrons that filter blood under high pressure, removing urea, salts, and other soluble wastes from